WHAT TO DO IN AN EMERGENCY

D0192480

IMMEDIATE TREATMENT

- Call out for someone to get help
- Look, listen, and feel for breathing (See p. 20.)
- Determine if the victim's heart is beating (See CPR, p. 22.)
- Stop excessive bleeding (See p. 80.)
- If something has been swallowed, ask victim what it was
- Treat for shock (See p. 234.)
- Perform the Heimlich maneuver for choking (See p. 36.)

WHAT TO TELL DOCTOR OR PARAMEDICS

- What has happened
- What the victim's noticeable injuries, symptoms, or signs are
- When the accident occurred or symptoms or signs began
- If known, what medications the victim has taken
- If poisoning has occurred, what has been swallowed, and when
- Where you and/or the victim are
- The phone number of your location
- Ask what more you can do to help

EMERGENCY TELEPHONE NUMBERS

Doctor _____

Doctor _____

Doctor _____

Ambulance _____

Police Department _____

Fire Department _____

Paramedics _____

Poison Control Center (local) _____

Hospital Emergency Room _____

Parents at Work _____

_____

Babysitter _____

Neighborhood Pharmacy _____

24-Hour Pharmacy _____

Electric Company _____

Gas Company _____

Neighbors _____

_____

_____

Relative _____

The American Medical Association Handbook of First Aid & Emergency Care

The American Medical Association

HANDBOOK

OF

FIRST AID

&

EMERGENCY

CARE

Developed by the American Medical Association

Medical Editors:
Stanley M. Zydlo, Jr., M.D.
Emergency Medicine
James A. Hill, M.D.
Sports Medicine

Illustrations by Larry Frederick

 RANDOM HOUSE   NEW YORK

Library of Congress Cataloging-in-Publication Data

American Medical Association.
    The American Medical Association handbook of first aid and emergency care/American Medical Association.—Rev. ed.
        p.   cm.
    Rev. ed. of: The American Medical Association handbook of first aid and emergency care. 1st ed. © 1980.
    ISBN 0-679-72959-3
    1. First aid in illness and injury—Popular works. 2. Medical emergencies—Popular works. I. American Medical Association. American Medical Association's handbook of first aid and emergency care. II. Title.
RC87.A535   1990
616.02'52—dc20   89-43545

CONTENTS

ABOUT THE
MEDICAL EDITORS

STANLEY M. ZYDLO, JR., M.D., is director of the Department of Emergency Medicine at Northwest Community Hospital in Arlington Heights, Illinois, and director of paramedic and emergency medical systems for both the city of Chicago and 22 northwest suburban communities. In addition, he is chairman of the board of Medical Emergency Service Associates (MESA), a professional corporation.

JAMES A. HILL, M.D., is associate professor of clinical orthopedic surgery at Northwestern Memorial Hospital in Chicago. He is also codirector of the Center for Sports Medicine at Northwestern University Medical School and, in 1988, served as the physician for the U.S. men's and women's basketball teams at the Olympics in Seoul, South Korea.

PREFACE

If a medical emergency were to strike you or a member of your family, would you be prepared to handle it? If a stranger collapsed in front of you, could you provide the necessary care required at a moment's notice? In a matter of seconds, and often without warning, you could be called upon to use your basic lifesaving skills to help someone in need.

In reality, we hope that you never have to use mouth-to-mouth resuscitation to help someone who has stopped breathing or CPR for a person whose heart has stopped beating. In cases in which you might have to, however, this book could be a lifesaver.

Our purpose in publishing this revised edition of the *AMA Handbook of First Aid and Emergency Care* is to help prepare you and members of your family for these and other emergency situations. Beyond the serious illnesses and injuries, we hope the *encouraging* message conveyed in this new edition is that many of the first-aid measures we learned as children and now use as adults simply require common sense: washing a wound on a scraped arm or leg, stopping minor bleeding with gentle pressure, or adding a kind word or extending a hand if someone has tripped or fallen. Your first reaction, instinctively, is oftentimes the correct one.

No one can stop accidents from occurring. When medical emergencies do occur—a heart attack, stroke, or choking—providing first aid within the crucial first few minutes can mean the difference between life and death. And when you perform first aid correctly, it enables paramedics and physicians to provide *their* care more effectively.

We hope that you will take the time now to read through and acquaint yourself with the procedures in this new edition so that it will serve you well in the event of an emergency.

We wish you continuing good health.

JAMES S. TODD, M.D.
Executive Vice President
American Medical Association

ACKNOWLEDGMENTS

Many individuals have given generously to the preparation of this book and we are indebted to all of them. In particular we would like to acknowledge the medical advisers and the editorial team who helped develop the original edition of this book: Gail V. Anderson, M.D. (Los Angeles); Christine E. Haycock, M.D. (Newark, N.J.); Stanley M. Zydlo, Jr., M.D. (Arlington Heights, Ill.); Martha Ross Franks (Midlothian, Va.); Charles C. Renshaw, Jr. (Chicago); Carole A. Fina (Phoenix); Sophie Klim (Chicago); and Marie Moore (Chicago).

We also wish to express our appreciation to Random House, Inc., particularly to Sam Vaughan, Janis Donnaud, Peter DeGiglio, and Olga Tarnowski, for their guidance and support in the preparation of this new edition of the book.

Also to Larry Frederick, whose illustrations appear within these pages, our appreciation for his fine work.

And, finally, a word of thanks to the AMA editorial team, whose creativity, skill, and dedication to excellence have been crucial to the quality of the manuscript: Kathleen A. Kaye, Brenda Clark, and Rita Castonguay.

HEIDI HOUGH
Director
American Medical Association
Office of Consumer Books

HOW TO LIVE
WITH THIS BOOK

USING THE AMA HANDBOOK OF FIRST AID AND EMERGENCY CARE

First-aid treatment in the first few minutes of an emergency can often mean the difference between life and death. Knowing what to do while reacting quickly and calmly before medical help arrives will enable you to provide the best care for the victim, whether it is you or someone else. In instances where an injury or illness is minor, knowing what to do and when to seek medical assistance can save needless telephone calls or visits to the doctor and unnecessary expense as well.

This book is designed to meet your immediate needs in emergency situations and to provide you with quick and easy access to this information. To help you find this information in an emergency, the book is divided into three parts.

READ NOW

Part I consists of general information that you should read *now*, before an emergency strikes. By reading these sections *now*, and by following the suggestions that are made and familiarizing yourself with certain methods and techniques, you will be better prepared to handle an emergency when it arises.

Part I has seven general information parts:

- Preparing for an Emergency—Now
- Safeguarding Your Home Against Accidents
- When to Call a Doctor
- Ambulance Services and Hospital Emergency Rooms
- Know Your Family's State of Health

- Techniques to Know and Use in Life/Death Situations
  - Cardiopulmonary Resuscitation (CPR)
  - Heimlich Maneuver (Abdominal Thrust)
- First-Aid Techniques to Learn and Practice

WHEN AN EMERGENCY ARISES

Part II is designed for quick, easy access at the time of an emergency and includes step-by-step treatment of specific injuries and illnesses. These injuries and illnesses, such as abdominal pain, broken bones, heart attack, stroke, and vomiting, are listed in alphabetical order so that you can find them quickly.

In case your name for an injury or an illness is different from ours, we have included a comprehensive index at the end of the book to ensure your quick access to the proper entry. Most of the alphabetical listings are organized with detailed *step-by-step* instructions. A few entries, however, such as Chills, Fever, Miscarriage, and Muscle Aches and Pains, provide *general information* about the subject, with recommendations on what you should do.

QUICK REFERENCE:
SPORTS FIRST AID

Finally, Part III of the book is an illustrated section with suggestions on treating 20 of the most common sports injuries, including runner's knee, tennis elbow, and swimmer's shoulder. This section appears on pages 265 to 319.

MEDICAL INSTRUCTIONS TO FOLLOW

To help point out and clarify the step-by-step medical instructions that you should follow in an emergency, certain terms are repeated throughout the alphabetical listing of entries. These terms are located to the left of the instructions. The meanings of these terms and how they appear are as follows:

ABCs
These letters refer to *a*irway, *b*reathing, and *c*irculation. They are the three basic steps in the procedure known as Cardiopulmonary Resuscitation (CPR). ABCs is a reminder to maintain an open airway and restore breathing and circulation, if necessary. (See the detailed description of CPR on p. 18).

The symbol and caption below will appear throughout the book to indicate a life-threatening situation.

ABCs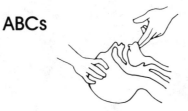

With all serious injuries, check and maintain an open *a*irway. Restore *b*reathing (p. 20) and *c*irculation (p. 22), if necessary.

Symptoms
A listing of certain conditions, such as pain, nausea, and swelling, that indicate a certain injury or illness may exist.

Immediate Treatment	Treatment for a serious condition, such as Choking, Third-Degree Burns, and Heart Attack, that you must begin *as soon as possible* before medical help arrives to prevent death or to decrease the severity of the problem.
Continued Care	Treatment that is begun only *after* the Immediate Treatment has been successfully carried out. Continued Care often includes prevention of shock and making the victim comfortable.
What to Do	Treatment for less serious injuries, such as scrapes, bruises, and blisters.
Danger Signals	A warning to seek medical attention promptly if symptoms continue or if other symptoms arise.

Other instructions that may appear include:

WARNING A warning that careful judgment and great care must be used with certain techniques, such as applying a tourniquet or rescuing a victim from drowning.

See also A cross-reference listing at the end of each entry that can provide you with additional information or refer you to another injury.

PART I

USING THE AMA HANDBOOK OF FIRST AID AND EMERGENCY CARE

PREPARING FOR AN EMERGENCY—NOW

MEDICAL CHART

One of the first things you should do is fill in, for each family member, the medical chart provided at the end of this book. The chart provides medical information you and doctors or paramedics need in an emergency, such as allergies and immunization dates. There is also a place for important emergency telephone numbers in the front of the book. *Fill these out now,* before you forget.

KNOW THE ROUTE TO THE HOSPITAL

Know the best route to the nearest hospital emergency room. If an ambulance or paramedic team is not available, you may have to drive yourself or a victim to the hospital. It is a good idea to make a practice run so that the roads will be familiar to you at the time of an emergency. Wrong turns can take precious minutes and could mean the difference between life and death.

EMERGENCY MEDICAL IDENTIFICATION

Wearing an emergency ID bracelet or necklace or carrying an emergency information card could save the life of someone who is unable to speak after a serious accident. This medical identification is particularly important for one who suffers from a serious condition such

3

as diabetes, epilepsy, glaucoma, or hemophilia, or who may have a serious allergic reaction to certain medications (such as penicillin) or to insect stings.

These bracelets, necklaces, and cards include such information as the individual's name, address, blood type, and any serious conditions or allergies. They should be worn or carried at all times. A bracelet or necklace is generally better than a card since it is more easily noticed on the victim. These items are available through several manufacturers. Ask your doctor, hospital emergency room, or local medical association where you might order them.

In the meantime, you can make your own card. Include your name, address, telephone number, name and telephone number of a relative to contact, your doctor's name and number, your immunization dates, any serious medical conditions, medication taken regularly, allergies, and any other important information. Be sure the card is prominently displayed in your purse or wallet.

SUPPLIES TO KEEP IN YOUR HOME AND CAR

Now is the time to assemble those basic items you may need when an injury or illness occurs in your home, car, boat, or while camping. Keep these items together in a box or other container and out of the reach of young children. Be sure to check the supplies periodically and replace used items. If a member of your family has special needs, ask your doctor what additional items you should include.

Keep on hand:

1. Roll of gauze bandage, 3 inches wide.
2. Sterile gauze pads packaged separately in sealed wrappers (nonstick type), 4 inches by 4 inches.
3. Bandages.
4. Butterfly bandages (tape) and thin adhesive strips, which hold skin edges together.
5. Roll of adhesive tape, 1-inch size.
6. Scissors.
7. A 3-inch elastic bandage (for wrapping sprained ankles and wrists).
8. Package of cotton-tipped swabs.
9. Roll of absorbent cotton (to be used as padding with a splint).

10. Aspirin (regular strength).
11. Acetaminophen, for pain relief (in liquid or tablet form for children under 16).
12. Oral and rectal thermometers.
13. Small jar of petroleum jelly to use with rectal thermometer.
14. Bottle of syrup of ipecac (to induce vomiting if poisons are swallowed).
15. Tweezers, without teeth.
16. Safety pins.
17. Small bottle of hydrogen peroxide (3-percent solution).
18. Calamine lotion.
19. Bar of plain soap.
20. Flashlight (particularly for car, boat, or when camping).
21. Snakebite kit (especially for camping).
22. An antihistamine, in liquid or tablet form, for allergic reactions.

EVERYDAY ITEMS THAT CAN BE USED IN AN EMERGENCY

Certain everyday items in your home—such as those listed below—can be used in an emergency. Keep in mind other items that may also be useful.

1. Disposable or regular diapers: to use as a compress to control heavy bleeding; for bandages; as padding for splints.
2. Sanitary napkins: to use as a compress to control heavy bleeding; for bandages; as padding for splints.
3. Towels, sheets, linens: to use as a compress to control heavy bleeding; for bandages; as padding for splints; in emergency childbirth.
4. Diaper pins: to use as pins for bandages or for a sling.
5. Blankets: to keep the victim warm.
6. Magazines, newspapers, umbrella, pillow: to use as splints for broken bones.
7. Table leaf, old door: to use as a stretcher for head, neck, and back injuries.
8. Fan: to cool the heatstroke victim.
9. Large scarf or handkerchief: to use as an eye bandage or a sling.

SAFEGUARDING YOUR HOME AGAINST ACCIDENTS

Keeping your home safe for you and your family should be your number-one health priority. Accidents, including those that occur in the home, are the fourth leading cause of death in the United States, according to the National Safety Council. Many of these deaths can be prevented.

To ensure that your home is safe, take a few minutes to read over the items listed below, and review them annually. The list is by no means all-inclusive. Other areas of the home to check regularly for safety hazards include closets, the attic, and additional storage areas such as outdoor pool and garden sheds.

One last reminder: Smoke detectors and fire extinguishers in your home are necessary investments and could save lives. Check them regularly and mark on a home calendar the date when batteries were last tested.

KITCHEN

1. Chemical cleaners: tightly capped or closed and properly stored out of the reach of children.
2. Liquor: properly stored out of the reach of children.
3. Knives: properly stored out of the reach of children.
4. Loose throw rugs: tacked down, held in place with carpet tape, or removed.
5. Frayed cords on electrical appliances: fixed or replaced.
6. Oven and stove top: cleaned regularly.
7. Refrigerator and freezer: cleaned and defrosted regularly.
8. Microwave oven: cleaned regularly and properly housed on a countertop or cart.
9. Other electrical appliances: cleaned and properly stored.

BATHROOM

1. Glass containers: removed or replaced with plastic containers.
2. Chemical cleaners: tightly capped or closed and properly stored out of the reach of children.

3. Electrical appliances (hair dryer, hair curling iron, electric shaver): unplugged and properly stored.
4. Old medicines in medicine cabinet: discarded. (If you wish to keep track of medications you or family members have taken, write them in the chart at the back of this book.)
5. Loose rugs or mats on floor: tacked down, held in place with carpet tape, or removed.
6. Tub and shower: adhesive grippers placed on the floor of the tub and railing along the wall to help prevent falls.

BASEMENT STAIRS

1. Broom, dustpan: stored on a rack on the wall or elsewhere.
2. Chemical cleaners: properly stored elsewhere.
3. Returnable bottles: returned or stored elsewhere.
4. Bags, boxes containing odds and ends: stored elsewhere.
5. Lighting: stairway adequately lit.

GARAGE OR BASEMENT

1. Cleaners and chemicals (rat poison and weed killers): tightly capped or closed and properly stored out of the reach of children.
2. Paint, paint thinners: tightly capped or closed and properly stored out of the reach of children. Throw out old paint.
3. Gasoline can: tightly closed and properly stored out of the reach of children.
4. Saws, chisels, other sharp blades: properly stored out of the reach of children.
5. Electric tools: unplugged, with safety locks on.
6. Old rags, old newspapers: discarded.
7. Loose cords, hoses: properly rolled up and stored.
8. Doors, windows, screens: properly stored.
9. Oil, gasoline spills: cleaned up.
10. Lighting: adequate throughout.
11. Buckets: emptied and properly stored. (Fluid-filled buckets are hazardous to infants and young children, who can drown in them.)

WHEN TO CALL A DOCTOR

At some time you may need to call a doctor about an injury or other medical problem. If the problem is a real emergency such as severe bleeding, a possible heart attack or stroke, a diabetic coma, or severe abdominal pain, call paramedics or an ambulance service to take the victim to the hospital.

If you are unsure of the victim's condition and the victim has severe or prolonged symptoms such as pain, vomiting and/or diarrhea (particularly with blood), difficulty in breathing, or high fever, call the victim's doctor—regardless of the hour.

It is very helpful when calling the doctor to give him or her specific information regarding the victim. Be prepared to tell the doctor or nurse the following:

- What has happened
- What the victim's noticeable injuries, symptoms, or signs are
- When the accident occurred or symptoms or signs began
- If known, what medications the victim has taken
- If poisoning has occurred, what has been swallowed, and when
- Where you and/or the victim are
- Give the phone number of your location
- Ask what more you can do to help

Above all else—and especially in an emergency situation—try to remain calm and follow the doctor's or medical professional's instructions. Your first-aid measures could save valuable seconds and, possibly, the life of the victim you are caring for.

AMBULANCE SERVICES AND HOSPITAL EMERGENCY ROOMS

It is necessary to call an ambulance to take a victim to a hospital emergency room anytime the victim's symptoms are critical or life-threatening—severe head, neck, or back injury, drug overdose, anaphylactic shock (shock caused by an allergic reaction to insect stings, medication, or food), or unconsciousness. In these instances the victim should be transported to the hospital as quickly as possible. If an ambulance is late or unavailable, *you* may have to drive the person to the hospital.

AMBULANCE SERVICES AND PARAMEDICS

Most communities have some type of ambulance service and specialized emergency medical personnel available. The most highly trained personnel are emergency medical technician–paramedics, or EMT-paramedics. They are trained to administer advanced life-support techniques along with cardiopulmonary resuscitation (CPR), to take electrocardiographic (ECG) tracings that reveal the electrical activity of the heart, and to give medication.

Other trained medical personnel can provide CPR and perform emergency medical procedures, such as splinting bones. Some can shock a victim's heart with specialized equipment if the heart has stopped beating. They cannot, however, administer medication or perform sophisticated medical procedures.

Many ambulances with paramedics have telemetry equipment hooked up to a local hospital that relays the electrocardiographic readings to the hospital and to physicians. Once the readings are received, a doctor's instructions can then be relayed to paramedics via radio.

Your community may have an ambulance service that provides transportation to the hospital but offers little or no emergency care. The attendants of such vehicles may not be trained to provide care beyond performing simple first aid.

Paramedics and other ambulance personnel are usually available through various community resources such as the fire department, police department, volunteer associations, and funeral homes. Check with the resources in your community before an emergency strikes so that you will know the type of service to call.

Paramedics should not be called for minor illnesses or injuries such as sprained ankles, minor cuts, or colds; they need to be available for people who have more serious conditions. Often victims with minor injuries can be driven to the hospital by a family member or friend.

WHEN TO GO TO THE EMERGENCY ROOM

It is difficult to answer the question "When should you go to the emergency room?" Anytime the victim's symptoms *appear* critical or life-threatening, he or she must be taken to the hospital. Any situation that *seems* like an emergency to you warrants a trip to the emergency room.

If you are taking someone to the hospital and there is time, call ahead to the emergency room or have someone else call. Tell them you are coming, the nature of the victim's injury or illness, and the name and phone number of the victim's doctor. This enables the emergency room staff to know what to expect, to prepare for the victim's arrival, and to contact the victim's doctor.

When the victim arrives at the hospital, he or she may be obliged to wait if the emergency room is busy, unless the victim's condition is serious or critical.

INFORMATION TO GIVE EMERGENCY ROOM PERSONNEL

The most serious and critical cases will be seen first. Any specific information you can give the emergency room staff about the victim's condition will help the staff determine its seriousness. Describing specific complaints, such as severe crushing chest pain or sharp lower abdominal pain, is very helpful. Other useful information includes:

1. When the symptoms began.
2. What makes the pain or condition better or worse.
3. What the victim was doing when the injury or illness occurred.
4. What changes have occurred to the victim since the onset of the illness or injury.
5. What—if anything—the victim has swallowed.
6. What medication the victim has been taking.

Certain other information about the victim will be needed by the hospital personnel. If time allows before leaving for the hospital, gather insurance identification cards, Medicare or Medicaid cards, or any other record of medical benefits to which the victim is entitled. Be prepared to give the victim's name, age, address, a history of major injuries or illnesses, and known allergies.

Laboratory tests and x-rays may be necessary. These tests aid in the investigative work of arriving at a diagnosis while initial treatment is being given.

Depending upon the size and the location of the hospital, most emergency rooms can offer full medical services ranging from bandaging a cut to surgery. If the emergency room cannot handle a specific situation, it must arrange to send the victim to another hospital that is capable of handling the medical problem.

Emergency room treatment is generally more expensive than medical treatment received in a doctor's office. Most emergency rooms must be staffed with doctors, nurses, and other personnel on a 24-hour basis, thus increasing their costs. Also, emergency rooms must be equipped with costly equipment not usually found in a doctor's office.

Most hospitals will process insurance forms. A number of hospitals are now also accepting major credit cards for payment.

KNOW YOUR FAMILY'S
STATE OF HEALTH

How do you know when you or someone in your family has a fever, rapid pulse, or dilated pupils? The best way is to be familiar with your family's normal state of health. Individual temperatures vary; a slight fever in one person may not indicate a fever in someone else. Remember: temperatures and pulse rates have different meanings for children and adults.

Temperature The average normal temperature taken by mouth is 98.6° Fahrenheit, plus or minus 1°. A Celsius thermometer, common in Canada and Europe, may be used instead of a Fahrenheit thermometer. An average normal temperature on a Celsius thermometer is 37°, plus or minus 1°.

An infant's temperature is taken rectally (with a rectal Fahrenheit or Celsius thermometer) and usually registers 1° higher than a normal oral temperature. (A temperature taken by mouth registers lower than a temperature taken rectally because air entering the mouth cools the mouth slightly, thus lowering the temperature *reading.*)

To find out what is normal for you, take your temperature when you know that you are not sick, at the same time of the day over a period of several days. Temperatures normally can vary 1° or more throughout the day. If your normal temperature varies slightly from the average, write it down next to your name on the medical chart at the back of this book, along with the date, so that everyone in the family will know what reading is normal for you. (See also the entry on Fever, p. 177, for additional information on high fevers and on how to take a temperature.)

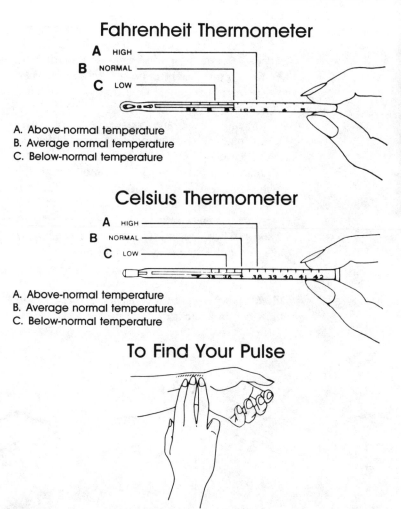

Fahrenheit Thermometer

A HIGH
B NORMAL
C LOW

A. Above-normal temperature
B. Average normal temperature
C. Below-normal temperature

Celsius Thermometer

A HIGH
B NORMAL
C LOW

A. Above-normal temperature
B. Average normal temperature
C. Below-normal temperature

To Find Your Pulse

To find your pulse, place three fingertips at your wrist just below the thumb.

Pulse Rate   The average normal pulse rate for an adult at rest is between 70 and 72 beats per minute. Individual pulse rates vary, of course, and can be slightly above or below the average. Well-conditioned athletes, for example, may have markedly lower pulse rates (50 to 60 beats per minute). Rates also can vary if you are excited or have just completed exercising or any other activity. To find your normal pulse rate, place three fingertips of one hand at your wrist just below the thumb on the palm side of your other hand. Count the pulsations for 60 seconds. Or, count for 15 seconds and multiply by 4. This is your pulse rate. Be sure to do this when you are rested and quiet, not after activity or emotional excitement.

Pulse rates in children vary according to age. The average pulse rate for a newborn infant is about 120 beats per minute. To find the pulse rate in infants, check below the left nipple or on the brachial artery (located on the inside of the arm between the elbow and the shoulder). A toddler's (1 to 5 years) pulse rate can be anywhere between 90 and 120 beats per minute. A child 5 to 15 years old has a pulse rate of between 70 and 100.

Pupils of the Eye

Pupils are the dark central portion of the eye. Dilated (very large) or constricted (very small) pupils can indicate a medical problem. To recog-

Changes in Pupil Size

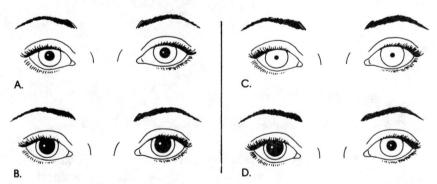

A.

C.

B.

D.

The pupils of the eye are located in the center of the iris.

A. Normal pupils (dark circles) are fairly small.
B. Dilated pupils (dark circles) are large and cover a large area of the iris.
C. Constricted pupils can be very small, about 1/16th of an inch in diameter.
D. Pupils that are unequal in size may indicate a serious medical condition and require prompt medical attention.

nize these conditions in yourself or someone else, you first need to know how normal pupils look. The best way to do this is to look at your own eyes in a mirror. Normal pupils are fairly small. Dilated pupils are quite large, while constricted pupils are like pinpoints, about 2 millimeters, or about 1/16th of an inch, in diameter.

Pupils that are noticeably different in size from one another can indicate a serious medical problem and may occur from a head injury, a stroke, or a previous eye injury. If you notice pupils that are unequal in size in yourself or in another person, seek prompt medical attention at a physician's office or hospital emergency room. (See Head and Neck Injuries, p. 188, and Stroke, p. 246.)

COMMON MEDICAL SYMPTOMS

There are several symptoms that all of us experience from time to time. The most common are fever, nausea, and headache. These symptoms may or may not indicate a serious medical condition.

Fever   is the body's way of indicating that something is wrong. Most often it indicates that an infection is present. A fever also may occur with asthma or allergies. In some cases, chills may precede a fever. (See Asthma, p. 61, Chills, p. 126, Croup, p. 88, Fever, p. 177, and Headaches, p. 187.)

Nausea   is a sick feeling in the stomach and is often accompanied by a desire to vomit. Nausea can be an early sign of pregnancy or a symptom of many disorders, such as excessive eating and drinking, allergic reactions to insect stings and spider or snake bites, drug withdrawal, reactions to medications, motion sickness, heart attack, heat exhaustion, food poisoning, fainting, vertigo, infections, appendicitis, and bowel obstruction. (See information for these conditions in Part II.)

Headaches   are most commonly caused by muscles tightening under the scalp, often the result of emotional tension. Other causes of headaches include infections, sinus infections, allergies, high blood pressure, multiple insect stings, head injuries, heat exhaustion, plant irritations, food poisoning, stroke, and brain tumor. They can also be danger signals in pregnancy. (See entries for these conditions in Part II.)

If a headache is accompanied by other symptoms, such as nausea, vomiting, a stiff neck, or visual disturbances (such as loss of vision, double vision, or blurred vision), seek immediate medical attention. (See Headaches, p. 187.)

ALARMING MEDICAL SYMPTOMS

Certain symptoms, such as convulsions in children and epileptic seizures, can be more frightening to experience or watch than dangerous to the victim. This does not mean, however, that you should ignore these conditions. All severe or prolonged symptoms should be reported to your doctor.

Certain other symptoms, such as the sudden onset of chest pain or the sudden loss of vision in one eye, indicate serious medical conditions. The victim should be transported without delay to a physician's office or to a hospital emergency room. At all times, try to remain calm so that your reaction does not frighten the victim.

Convulsions (seizures) in children are most commonly caused by a rapid rise in temperature due to an acute infection. These convulsions (called febrile convulsions) seldom last longer than two to three minutes. (If the convulsions last longer, seek immediate medical treatment at a hospital emergency room.) All febrile convulsions should be reported to your doctor.

Another common type of convulsion is an *epileptic seizure,* which usually occurs in people who have a hereditary tendency to have convulsions. However, epileptic seizures may occur for unknown reasons. The seizures occur when some brain cells temporarily become overactive and release too much electrical energy, stimulating part or all of the brain. The primary aim of the first-aider is to prevent the victim from harming himself or herself. Contrary to myth, a person having a seizure is not in danger of biting off or swallowing his or her tongue. Do *not* put any object into the victim's mouth. After the seizure is over, consult the victim's doctor. (See Convulsions, p. 133.)

Headaches are a very common complaint. But the sudden onset of a **severe headache** with nausea, vomiting, or visual disturbances, or in conjunction with a stiff neck, requires immediate medical attention. A severe headache of this kind may be symptomatic of meningitis, encephalitis, stroke, or a tumor. (See Headaches, p. 187.)

Sudden, unexpected **loss of consciousness** may mean that the victim has suffered a stroke or a heart attack, or has stopped breathing. He or she may require cardiopulmonary resuscitation (CPR). Refer to information on ABCs—clearing *a*irway, restoring *b*reathing, and restoring *c*irculation—on pages 19 through 35. (See also Unconsciousness, p. 251.)

Sudden, unexpected onset of **severe chest pain** may signal a heart attack and is a life-threatening emergency. (See Heart Attack, p. 196.)

Sudden, unexpected **loss of vision in one eye** may be the onset of a stroke. Seek medical attention for the victim immediately. (See Stroke, p. 246.)

Sudden **loss of sensation or motion in an extremity** (arm or leg) may result from a stroke or a brain tumor. The condition should be brought to the attention of a physician without delay. Do not wait until the symptom goes away. Even if the symptom *does* disappear, seek medical attention. (See Stroke, p. 246.)

Shortness of breath   for no apparent reason may mean the onset of an asthma attack or an acute allergic reaction, or may be symptomatic of congestive heart failure. Seek medical attention immediately to rule out a serious medical condition. (See also Asthma, p. 61.)

The presence of **blood in the urine** may signal an infection, or, more seriously, a malignancy. The presence of **blood in the stool** (black stool) or with a bowel movement may signal an ulcer or bowel or stomach cancer. These symptoms require immediate medical attention. (See Bleeding, p. 80.)

TECHNIQUES TO KNOW
AND USE IN LIFE/DEATH
SITUATIONS

Basic lifesaving skills that you should become familiar with *and stay familiar with* are cardiopulmonary resuscitation (CPR) and—in cases in which a victim is choking—the Heimlich maneuver (abdominal thrust). Information on CPR follows below. Instructions for the Heimlich maneuver begin on page 36.

NOTE: *Do not use either procedure on individuals who are not in distress.*

CARDIOPULMONARY RESUSCITATION (CPR)*

CPR is a basic life-support technique used when the victim is not breathing and it is possible that his or her heart has stopped beating. The technique allows you to perform manually the involuntary actions of the heart and lungs that provide vital blood and oxygen to all parts of the body.

*NOTE: There is concern among those who provide first aid—even on a onetime basis—that AIDS may be contracted from a victim's body fluids. It is *extremely unlikely* that you—as a first-aider providing emergency care—will contract AIDS from a victim who is bleeding or from the saliva of a victim who may require mouth-to-mouth resuscitation or CPR.

AIDS is present in individuals who have been infected with HIV—human immunodeficiency virus. The infection, caused by the virus, weakens the body's immune system, rendering the individual "immune-deficient." Over time, the body becomes unable to fight off disease.

AIDS can be passed to others through an infected person's blood and semen. The AIDS virus may be present in saliva, but cases in which AIDS has been transmitted through saliva are unknown at the present time.

You may be aware that those *who regularly come in contact with a patient's or victim's blood or saliva*—doctors, paramedics, other emergency room personnel, and dentists—have begun wearing protective face masks and gloves. *Even among these health-care professionals, the risk of contracting AIDS is very low.*

CPR involves opening and clearing the victim's *a*irway (by tilting the head backward and lifting the chin), restoring *b*reathing (by mouth-to-mouth, mouth-to-nose, or mouth-to-mouth-and-nose resuscitation), and restoring blood *c*irculation (by external chest compressions). Although opening the victim's airway and restoring breathing can be done effectively at the time of the crisis by following the instructions in this book, restoring circulation with manual chest compressions—also outlined in this book—*should be learned through classroom instruction taught by qualified personnel* to be most effective. Additionally, regular practice and refresher courses are recommended. (If your community does not offer a course in CPR, call your local Heart Association or the American Red Cross for information.)

ABC A simple method of remembering the order of action to take in an emergency if the victim is not breathing or if his or her heart is not beating is the use of the term "ABCs." These letters stand for *a*irway, *b*reathing, and *c*irculation. They are the three basic steps in the procedure known as cardiopulmonary resuscitation (CPR).

ABCs

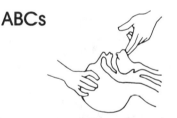

With all serious injuries, check and maintain an open *a*irway. Restore *b*reathing (p. 20) and *c*irculation (p. 22), if necessary.

(A) Airway

The victim's airway must be clear and open, in order to restore breathing.

Clear the airway by doing the following:

1. Lay the victim on his or her back on a firm, rigid surface such as the floor or the ground. For an infant, the hard surface may be the palm of the hand.

2. Quickly clear the mouth and airway of foreign material with your fingers.
3. If there does not appear to be any neck injury,* tilt the head backward to open the airway. Do this by placing your palm on the victim's forehead and the fingers of your other hand under the bony part of the victim's chin. Doing this will elevate the tongue from the back of the throat.

    For an infant or small child, tilt the head back only slightly, so that the airway does not become closed off.

(B) Breathing

To restore breathing:

1. Be sure that the victim's head is tilted backward.
2. With the hand that is placed on the victim's forehead, pinch the victim's nostrils closed, using your thumb and index finger.
3. Open your mouth widely and take a deep breath.
4. Place your open mouth tightly around the victim's mouth and give 2 full breaths—so that air enters his or her lungs—1 to 1½ seconds per breath. Remove your mouth after each of your exhalations and take a deep breath between each of your breaths.

    For an infant or small child, place your mouth tightly over the victim's mouth and nose. Use less air for an infant.
5. If the victim's mouth cannot be used due to an injury, lift the lower jaw to close the mouth. Open your mouth wide and take a deep breath. Place your mouth tightly around the victim's nose and blow into it. After your exhale, remove your hand from the victim's mouth to allow air to escape.
6. Moderate resistance will be felt when you blow. If you encounter *marked* resistance and the chest does not rise, the airway is not clear and more airway opening is needed. Place your hands under the victim's lower jaw and thrust the lower jaw forward so that it juts out farther.
7. As you blow air into the victim's mouth, nose, or mouth and

---

*In cases in which you suspect a head or neck injury, especially if the victim has fallen from a height, has fallen from a motorcycle, has been hit by a car, or has been involved in a diving accident, *and* if he or she is unconscious, *do not* move the victim. (See Head and Neck Injuries, p. 188.)

Exceptions to this rule would occur when you and the victim are in imminent danger of death, such as in or near a fire, at an accident scene in which an explosion might occur, or near a collapsing building.

Mouth-to-Mouth Resuscitation

If the victim is not breathing:

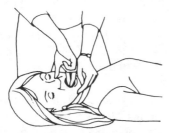

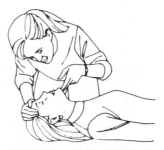

1. Make sure the victim is on a hard, flat surface. Quickly clear the mouth and airway of foreign material.

2. Tilt the victim's head backward by placing the palm of your hand on his or her forehead and the fingers of your other hand under the bony part of the chin.

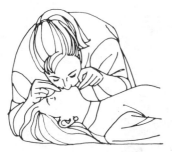

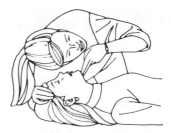

3. Pinch the victim's nostrils with your thumb and index finger. Take a deep breath. Place your mouth tightly over the victim's mouth (mouth and nose for an infant or small child). Give 2 quick breaths.

4. Stop blowing when the chest is expanding. Remove your mouth from the victim's mouth and turn your head toward the victim's chest, so that your ear is over his or her mouth. *Listen* for air being exhaled. *Watch* for the victim's chest to fall. Repeat the breathing procedure.

nose, watch closely to see when his or her chest rises, and stop blowing when the chest is expanding.

8. Remove your mouth from the victim's mouth, nose, or mouth and nose and turn your head toward the victim's chest so that your ear is over his or her mouth. Listen for air leaving the victim's lungs and watch the chest fall. You may also feel air being exhaled from the victim's nose and mouth.

9. Continue blowing into the victim's mouth, nose, or mouth and nose at approximately 12 breaths per minute (1 breath every 5 seconds) for an adult; 15 breaths per minute (1 breath every 4 seconds) for a child; and 20 breaths per minute (1 breath every 3 seconds) for an infant. Quantity is important, so provide plenty of air with each breath so that the victim's chest rises.
10. Continue breathing for the victim until he or she begins breathing on his or her own or until medical assistance arrives.
11. If a drowning victim's stomach is bloated with swallowed water, put the victim on his or her stomach with the head turned to the side. To empty water, place both hands under the victim's stomach and lift. After water is emptied, or if no water is emptied after approximately ten seconds, return the victim to his or her back. Resume mouth-to-mouth breathing until the victim is breathing well on his or her own or until medical assistance arrives.

To Aid a Drowning Victim

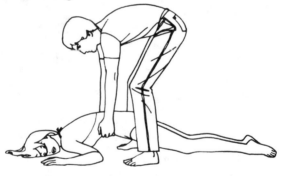

To remove water from a victim's stomach, place both hands under the stomach and lift.

(C) Circulation

To restore blood circulation: This is best done by those professionally trained and *must* be done in conjunction with artificial breathing. In emergency situations, however, restoring circulation for the victim is essential for survival, and chest compressions, as outlined below, should be attempted. If you are performing CPR, have someone else call paramedics or an ambulance.

The information below includes steps for clearing the airway and restoring breathing that have been discussed previously.

To Perform CPR for an Adult:

First:

1. Assess the situation. Is the victim conscious? Gently shake him or her and shout: "Are you okay?"
2. If there is no response, call to someone to get help.
3. *Look, listen,* and *feel* for breathing. Look for the victim's chest to rise and fall.
4. Check for any foreign matter in the mouth. If the victim is not breathing, tilt the head backward to open the airway. Do this by placing your palm on the victim's forehead and the fingers of your other hand under the bony part of the victim's chin.
5. Pinch the victim's nose closed and blow 2 full breaths into his or her mouth so that the chest rises. Remove your mouth after each of your exhalations and take a deep breath between each of your breaths.

To Find a Pulse

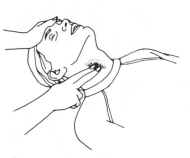

To check for a pulse on the victim's neck (carotid artery): move two fingers along the victim's throat to the Adam's apple. Then move these fingers off to the side of the victim's throat between the trachea (windpipe) and the muscles at the side of the neck. Press down gradually and firmly until you feel a pulse. *A pulse means that the heart is beating.*

6. With the palm of one hand on the victim's forehead (to ensure that the head is tilted backward and that the airway is open), with the other hand check for a pulse on the victim's neck (carotid artery). To find the pulse in the carotid artery, move two fingers along the victim's throat to the Adam's apple. Then move these fingers off to the side of the victim's throat between the trachea (windpipe) and the muscles at the side of the neck. Press down gradually and firmly until you feel a pulse. *A pulse means that the heart is beating.*

7. If there is a pulse, but no breathing, perform mouth-to-mouth resuscitation at 12 breaths per minute—1 breath every 5 seconds. (See p. 20.)
8. If there is no pulse, begin chest compressions as well. (See below.)

To establish proper hand position for chest compressions:

(**NOTE:** *Proper hand position is important so that you do not damage ribs or internal organs.*)

1. If possible, make sure that the victim is lying on a hard, flat surface. The head should be at the same level as the rest of the body or slightly lower so that blood flow to the brain is not further reduced. If possible, slightly elevate the legs, which will help blood flow back to the heart. *Move quickly, however, so that valuable time is not lost.*
2. Kneel near the victim's chest. With two fingers, locate the victim's rib cage on the side closest to you.
3. Move your fingers up the center of the victim's chest to the notch where the ribs meet the breastbone (sternum).

Hand Position for CPR

Move your fingers up the center of the victim's chest to the notch where the ribs meet the breastbone (sternum). With two fingers on this notch, place the heel of your other hand two finger-widths above your fingers. Remove your fingers from the notch and place this hand on top of your other hand. The fingers may be interlaced. Do not allow your fingers to rest on the ribs.

4. With your fingers on this notch, place the heel of your other hand two finger-widths above your fingers.
5. Remove your fingers from the notch and place this hand on top of your other hand. The fingers may be interlaced.

To Perform Chest Compressions

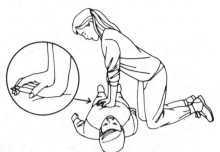

After finding the correct hand position for CPR (see previous page), push down on the chest 15 times. With each compression, push down quickly and forcefully to a depth of 1½ to 2 inches. Let the chest rise after each compression, *but do not remove your hands from the chest.*

6. Do not allow your fingers to rest on the ribs. Press down with the heel of your hand only.
7. While kneeling, position your shoulders directly over the victim so that all of your weight is forced down, through the heel of your hand, onto the victim's chest. Straighten your arms and lock your elbows. Use your arms as pistons to exert pressure.

To perform compressions:

1. Push down on the chest 15 times. With each compression, push down quickly and forcefully to a depth of 1½ to 2 inches. Let the chest rise after each compression, *but do not remove your hands from the chest.*
2. Perform this technique rhythmically by counting out loud: "*one* and, *two* and, *three* and, *four* and, *five* and, *six* and, *seven* and, *eight* and, *nine* and, *ten* and, *eleven* and, *twelve* and, *thirteen* and, *fourteen* and, *fifteen* and."
3. Release your hands from the victim's chest and open the airway by tilting the head and chin backward.
4. Pinch the victim's nostrils shut with your thumb and index finger. Blow 2 full breaths into the victim's mouth so that the chest rises.
5. Reposition your hands on the victim's chest and repeat the 15 compressions and 2 breaths.

6. Perform 4 complete cycles of 15 compressions and 2 breaths. Then, determine if the victim's pulse has returned. To do this, feel the victim's carotid artery in the neck. *Do not, however, interrupt CPR for longer than 7 seconds.*

7. To find the pulse in the carotid artery, move two fingers along the victim's throat to the Adam's apple. Then move these fingers off to the side of the victim's throat between the trachea (windpipe) and the muscles at the side of the neck. Press down gradually and firmly until you feel a pulse. *A pulse means that the heart is beating.*

8. *If there is a pulse but no breathing, perform mouth-to-mouth resuscitation, at 12 breaths per minute—1 breath every 5 seconds. (See p. 20.)*

9. *If there is no pulse, repeat the 15 compressions and 2 breaths.*

10. Continue CPR until the victim begins breathing and his or her heart begins beating, until professional help arrives, or until you are too tired to continue.

11. *If vomiting occurs during CPR,* turn the victim on his or her side (rolling the victim's whole body as a unit) and clear out the mouth with your fingers. Return the victim to his or her back and tilt the head backward to open the airway. Resume mouth-to-mouth resuscitation and CPR if necessary.

To Perform CPR for a Child (8 Years or Younger):

(For large children or for those over age 8, use the steps outlined for an adult.)

First:

1. Assess the situation. Is the victim conscious? Gently shake him or her and shout: "Are you okay?"

2. If there is no response, call to someone to get help.

3. *Look, listen,* and *feel* for breathing. Look for the victim's chest to rise and fall.

4. Check for any foreign matter in the mouth. If the victim is not breathing, tilt the head backward to open the airway. Do this by placing your palm on the victim's forehead and the fingers of your other hand under the bony part of the victim's chin.

5. Place your mouth over the victim's mouth and nose and blow 2 full breaths so that the victim's chest rises. Remove your mouth after each of your exhalations and take a deep breath between each of your breaths.

Mouth-to-Mouth-and-Nose Resuscitation

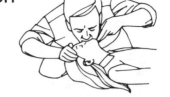

To breathe air into the victim's lungs: Place your mouth over the victim's mouth and nose and blow 2 full breaths so that his or her chest rises. Take a deep breath between each of your breaths.

6. With the palm of one hand on the victim's forehead (to ensure that the head is tilted backward and that the airway is open), with the other hand check for a pulse on the victim's neck (carotid artery). To find the pulse in the carotid artery, move two fingers along the victim's throat to the Adam's apple. Then move these fingers off to the side of the victim's throat, between the trachea (windpipe) and the muscles at the side of the neck. Press down gradually and firmly until you feel a pulse. *A pulse means that the heart is beating.*

To Find a Pulse

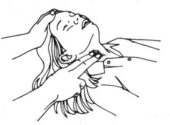

To check for a pulse on the victim's neck (carotid artery): Move two fingers along the victim's throat to the Adam's apple. Then move these fingers off to the side of the victim's throat between the trachea (windpipe) and the muscles at the side of the neck. Press down gradually and firmly until you feel a pulse. *A pulse means that the heart is beating.*

7. If there is a pulse but no breathing, perform mouth-to-mouth-and-nose resuscitation at 15 breaths per minute (1 breath every 4 seconds). (See p. 20.)
8. If there is no pulse, begin chest compressions as well. (See below.)

To establish proper hand position for chest compressions:

(**NOTE:**   *Proper hand position is important so that you do not damage ribs or internal organs.*)

1.   If possible, make sure that the victim is lying on a hard, flat surface. The head should be at the same level as the rest of the body or slightly lower so that blood flow to the brain is not further reduced. If possible, slightly elevate the legs, which will help blood flow back to the head. *Move quickly, however, so that valuable time is not lost.*
2.   Kneel near the victim's chest. With two fingers, locate the victim's rib cage on the side closest to you.
3.   Move your fingers up the center of the victim's chest to the notch where the ribs meet the breastbone (sternum).
4.   With your fingers on this notch, place the heel of your other hand next to and above your fingers.
5.   Remove your fingers from the notch. Use one hand only for compressions.

Hand Position for CPR

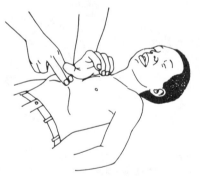

Move your fingers up the center of the victim's chest to the notch where the ribs meet the breastbone (sternum). With your fingers on this notch, place the heel of your other hand two finger-widths above your fingers. Remove your fingers from the notch. Use one hand only for compressions.

6.   Do not let your fingers rest on the ribs. Press down with the heel of your hand only.
7.   While kneeling, position your shoulders directly over the victim so that all of your weight is forced down, through the heel of

your hand, onto the victim's chest. Straighten your arm and lock your elbow. Use your arm as a piston to exert pressure.

To perform compressions:

1. Push down on the chest 5 times. With each compression push down quickly and forcefully to a depth of 1 to 1½ inches. Let the chest rise after each compression, *but do not remove your hand from the chest.*
2. Perform this technique rhythmically by counting out loud: "*one* and, *two* and, *three* and, *four* and, *five* and."

To Perform Chest Compressions

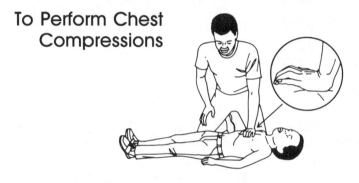

After finding the correct hand position for CPR (see previous page), push down on the chest 5 times. With each compression push down quickly and forcefully to a depth of 1 to 1½ inches. Let the chest rise after each compression, *but do not remove your hand from the chest.*

3. Release your hand from the victim's chest and open the airway by tilting the head and chin backward.
4. Blow 1 full breath into the victim's mouth and nose so that the chest rises.
5. Reposition your hand on the victim's chest and repeat the 5 compressions and 1 breath.
6. Perform 10 complete cycles of 5 compressions and 1 breath. Then, determine if the victim's pulse has returned. To do this, feel the victim's carotid artery in the neck. *Do not, however, interrupt CPR for longer than 7 seconds.*
7. To find the pulse in the carotid artery, move two fingers along the victim's throat to the Adam's apple. Then move these fingers off to the side of the victim's throat between the trachea (windpipe) and the muscles at the side of the neck. Press down

gradually and firmly until you feel a pulse. *A pulse means that the heart is beating.*

8. *If there is a pulse, but no breathing, perform mouth-to-mouth-and-nose resuscitation at 15 breaths per minute (1 breath every 4 seconds). (See p. 20.)*

9. *If there is no pulse, repeat the 5 compressions and 1 breath.*

10. Continue CPR until the victim begins breathing and his or her heart begins beating, until professional help arrives, or until you are too tired to continue.

11. *If vomiting occurs during CPR,* turn the victim on his or her side (rolling the victim's whole body as a unit) and clear out the mouth with your fingers. Return the victim to his or her back and tilt the head backward to open the airway. Resume mouth-to-mouth-and-nose resuscitation and CPR if necessary.

To Perform CPR for an Infant:

First:

1. Assess the situation. Is the infant conscious? Gently shake him or her and shout, "Are you okay?" to elicit a cry or other response.

2. If there is no response, call to someone to get help.

3. *Look, listen,* and *feel* for breathing. Look for the infant's chest to rise and fall.

Mouth-to-Mouth-and-Nose Resuscitation

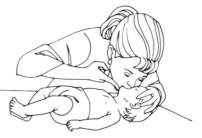

To breathe air into an infant's lungs: Place your mouth over the infant's mouth and nose and blow 2 breaths so that his or her chest rises. Do not blow air as forcefully as for an adult. Take a breath between each of your breaths.

4. Check for any foreign matter in the mouth. If the infant is not breathing, tilt the head backward to open the airway. Do this by placing your palm on the infant's forehead and the fingers of your other hand under the bony part of the infant's chin. *Do not extend the head too far back. Doing so may close off the airway.*

5. Place your mouth over the infant's mouth and nose and blow 2 breaths so that his or her chest rises. Do not blow air as forcefully as for an adult. Remove your mouth after each of your exhalations and take a breath between each of your breaths.

6. With the palm of one hand on the infant's forehead (to ensure that the head is tilted backward and that the airway is open), with the other hand check for a pulse in the infant's brachial artery, located on the inside of the upper arm between the elbow and shoulder. *A pulse means that the heart is beating.*

To Find a Pulse

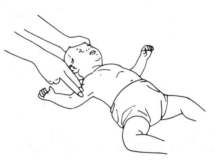

Check for a pulse on the infant's brachial artery, located on the inside of the upper arm between the elbow and shoulder. *A pulse means that the heart is beating.*

7. If there is a pulse but no breathing, perform mouth-to-mouth-and-nose resuscitation at 20 breaths per minute (1 breath every 3 seconds). (See p. 20.)

8. If there is no pulse, begin chest compressions as well. (See below.)

To establish proper finger position on the chest for CPR:

(**NOTE:** *Proper finger position is important so that you do not damage ribs or internal organs.*)

1. If possible, place the infant on his or her back on a hard, flat surface. The head should be at the same level as the rest of the

body or slightly lower so that blood flow to the brain is not further reduced. *Move quickly, however, so that valuable time is not lost.*

2. Place the palm of your hand on the infant's forehead and tilt the head back. *Do not extend the head too far back. Doing so may close off the airway.*

3. With your other hand, locate an imaginary line between the infant's nipples on the breastbone.

4. Place two fingers one finger-width below this line on the breastbone.

Finger Position for CPR

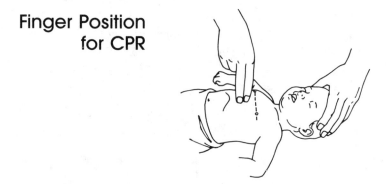

Locate an imaginary line between the infant's nipples on the breastbone. Place two fingers one finger-width below this line on the breastbone.

5. Try to keep your palm in position on the infant's forehead and your fingers in position on the infant's chest throughout compressions. (You may find it easier to steady the infant's head and body during compressions by placing your fingers and thumb on either side of the infant's head. See illustration.)

To perform compressions:

1. Using two fingers, push down on the chest 5 times. With each compression, push down to a depth of ½ to 1 inch. Let the chest rise after each compression, *but do not remove your fingers from the chest.*

2. Perform this technique rhythmically by counting out loud: "*one* and, *two* and, *three* and, *four* and, *five* and."

3. After 5 compressions, blow air once into the infant's mouth and nose.

CPR Dos and Don'ts

The success of your CPR efforts will depend in large part on performing the CPR technique properly. Below is a list of reminders to help you. Remember: Perform CPR only if you do not feel a pulse.

Do	Don't
1. Kneel alongside the victim to perform chest compressions. Straighten your arms and lock your elbows. Use your arms as pistons to exert pressure.	1. Rock back and forth or sit on your heels while performing compressions. (Blood will not be pumped out of the heart effectively.)
2. Perform quick, forceful compressions straight down on the chest.	2. Roll your hands on the chest.
3. Keep your hands in place on the chest while performing compressions.	3. Lift your hands off the chest or "bounce" your hands on the chest while performing compressions.
4. Interlock fingers and use the heel of one hand only for compressions.	4. Allow the fingers to rest or exert pressure on the rib cage.

4. Perform 10 complete cycles of 5 compressions and 1 breath. Then, determine if the infant's pulse has returned. To do this, feel for a pulse in the brachial artery, located on the inside of the upper arm between the elbow and shoulder. *A pulse means that the heart is beating. Do not, however, interrupt CPR for longer than 7 seconds.*

5. *If there is a pulse but no breathing, perform mouth-to-mouth-and-nose resuscitation at 20 breaths per minute (1 breath every 3 seconds). (See p. 20.)*

6. *If there is no pulse, repeat the 5 compressions and 1 breath.*

7. Continue CPR until the infant begins breathing and his or her heart begins beating, until professional help arrives, or until you are too tired to continue.

8. *If vomiting occurs during CPR,* turn the infant on his or her side, and clear out the mouth with your fingers. Return the infant to

CPR Reminders

	Adults	Children	Infants
If there is a **pulse but no breathing,** give 1 breath every:	5 seconds (12 per minute)	4 seconds (15 per minute)	3 seconds (20 per minute)
If there is **no pulse,** begin CPR by:	Tracing the ribs to the notch at the center of the chest. Place the heel of the other hand 2 finger-widths above the notch.	*Same as adult*	Placing 2 fingers one finger-width below the nipple line.
Push down on (compress) the chest with:	The heel of one hand on the breastbone, with the other hand on top of it.	The heel of one hand only on the breastbone.	2 or 3 fingers on the breastbone.
Compress the chest to a depth of:	1½–2 inches	1–1½ inches	½–1 inch
Number of compressions to breaths:	15:2	5:1	5:1

his or her back and tilt the head backward to open the airway. Resume mouth-to-mouth-and-nose resuscitation and CPR if necessary.

Glossary of CPR Terms

ABCs
A term that describes the three basic components of CPR: maintain an open airway, restore breathing, and restore circulation, if necessary.

Brachial artery
One of the main arteries in the body, found on the inside of the upper arm, between the elbow and shoulder. A rescuer can feel for a pulse—primarily in infants—by gently, but firmly, pressing on this artery.

Cardiac arrest
A critical medical condition in which the heart has stopped beating.

CPR
Cardiopulmonary resuscitation. Literally, heart and lung revival. The process of clearing the airway, restoring breathing, and restoring blood circulation.

Carotid artery
One of the main arteries in the body, found on either side of the neck. A rescuer can feel for a pulse—primarily in children and adults—by gently, but firmly, pressing on this artery.

Compressions
Downward thrusts on the chest with the hands. Compressing or pushing down on the chest, like pressing down on a sponge, pushes blood out of the heart to all parts of the body. Releasing pressure on the chest allows the rib cage to expand and, again similar to the dynamics of a sponge, draws blood into the heart.

Pulse
The "wave" of blood flowing through arteries and veins that is in rhythm with the beating of the heart. When a rescuer feels for a pulse in one of the main arteries in the body, he or she is determining if the heart is beating.

Respiration
The process of breathing.

Resuscitation
The attempt to restore breathing and, if necessary, blood circulation in a victim. This is done by mouth-to-mouth, mouth-to-nose, or mouth-to-

	mouth-and-nose respirations and by chest compressions.
Ventilations	The process of breathing air into a victim's lungs. This is done in mouth-to-mouth, mouth-to-nose, or mouth-to-mouth-and-nose resuscitation.

HEIMLICH MANEUVER (ABDOMINAL THRUST)

The Heimlich maneuver (abdominal thrust) is the method of choice to use in an emergency situation when a person is choking. Back blows—hitting the victim forcefully and repeatedly between the shoulder blades with the palm of your hand—are used on adults and children only if the Heimlich maneuver has not been effective in dislodging a foreign object from the windpipe (trachea).

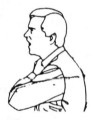

The Universal Choking Sign

A person who is choking will involuntarily grasp his or her neck.

Heimlich Maneuver

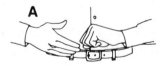

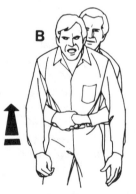

B

A. Correct placement of fist with thumb side against victim's stomach slightly above the navel and below the ribs and breastbone.
B. If victim is standing or sitting, stand behind victim with your arms around his or her waist. Place your fist as shown in illustration. Hold your fist with your other hand and give 4 quick, forceful upward thrusts.

Heimlich Maneuver on a Child

Stand behind the child with your arms around his or her waist. Place the thumb side of your fist against the child's stomach slightly above the navel and below the ribs and breastbone. Hold your fist with your other hand and give 4 quick, forceful upward thrusts. It may be necessary to repeat the procedure 6 to 10 times.

For an Adult or a Child:

If the Victim Is Conscious:

1. If the victim can speak, cough, or breathe (meaning that he or she is moving air through the airway), do not interfere in any way with his or her efforts to cough out a swallowed or partially swallowed object.
2. If the victim cannot breathe, stand behind him or her and place your fist with the thumb side against the victim's stomach slightly above the navel and below the ribs and breastbone. Hold your fist with your other hand and give 4 quick, forceful upward thrusts. This maneuver increases pressure in the abdomen, which pushes up the diaphragm. This, in turn, increases the air pressure in the lungs and will often force out the object from the windpipe.

    Do not squeeze on the ribs with your arms. Just use your fist in the abdomen. It may be necessary to repeat the Heimlich maneuver 6 to 10 times.
3. If the victim is lying down, turn the victim on his or her back. Straddle the victim and put the heel of your hand on the victim's stomach, slightly above the navel and below the ribs. Put your free hand on top of your other hand to provide additional force.

Heimlich Maneuver on a Victim Lying Down

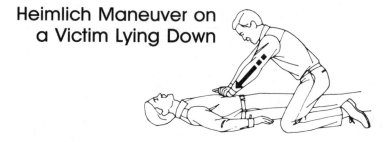

Straddle the victim and put the heel of your hand on the victim's stomach, slightly above the navel and below the ribs. Put your free hand on top of your other hand. Keep your elbows straight. Give 4 quick, forceful downward and forward thrusts toward the head.

Keep your elbows straight. Give 4 quick, forceful downward and forward thrusts toward the head in an attempt to dislodge the object. Doing so will increase pressure in the abdomen, forcing pressure into the lungs to expel the object out of the windpipe and into the mouth.

It may be necessary to repeat the procedure 6 to 10 times.

4. If you get no results, repeat the Heimlich maneuver until the victim coughs up the object or becomes unconscious. Look to see if the object appears in the victim's mouth or the top of the throat. Use your fingers to pull the object out.

If the Victim Is Unconscious or Becomes Unconscious:

1. Place the victim on his or her back on a rigid surface, such as the ground.
2. Open the victim's airway by extending the head backward. To do this, place the palm of your hand on the victim's forehead and the fingers of your other hand under the bony part of the chin. Attempt to restore breathing with mouth-to-mouth resuscitation. (See p. 20.)
3. If still unsuccessful, and with the victim on his or her back, begin the Heimlich maneuver by putting the heel of one hand on the victim's stomach slightly above the navel and below the ribs. Put your free hand on top of your other hand to provide additional force. Keep your elbows straight. Give 4 quick, forceful, downward and forward thrusts toward the head.
4. If these procedures fail, grasp the victim's lower jaw and tongue with one hand and lift up to remove the tongue from the back

of the throat. Place the index finger of the other hand inside the victim's mouth alongside the cheek. Slide your fingers down into the throat to the base of the victim's tongue.

Carefully sweep your fingers along the back of the throat to dislodge the object. Bring your fingers out along the inside of the other cheek. Be careful not to push the object farther down the victim's throat. If a foreign body comes within reach, grasp and remove it. *Do not* attempt to remove the foreign object with any type of instrument or forceps unless you are trained to do so.

5. Repeat all of the above steps until the object is dislodged or medical assistance arrives. Do not give up!

If the Victim Is an Infant:

1. Place the infant face down across your forearm with his or her head low. Support the head by firmly holding the jaw.

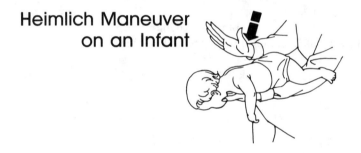

Heimlich Maneuver on an Infant

Rest your forearm on your thigh. Support the infant's head by firmly holding the jaw. Give 4 forceful back blows with the heel of your hand between the infant's shoulder blades. If unsuccessful, turn the infant over and give 4 quick thrusts on the chest. To do this, place 2 fingers one finger-width below an imaginary line joining the nipples. Push downward and forward. Thrusts should be more gentle than those for an adult. Repeat both procedures if necessary.

2. Rest your forearm on your thigh and give 4 forceful back blows with the heel of your hand between the infant's or child's shoulder blades. The blows should be more gentle than those for an adult.

3. If unsuccessful, turn the infant over and give 4 quick thrusts on the chest. To do this, place 2 fingers one finger-width below an

imaginary line joining the nipples. Push downward and forward. Thrusts should be more gentle than those for an adult.

4.   If necessary, repeat both procedures.

If the Victim Is Very Fat or Is Pregnant:

1.   Stand behind the victim and place your fist on the middle of the breastbone in the chest, but not over the ribs. Put your other hand on top of it. Give 4 quick, forceful movements. *Do not* squeeze with your arms. Just use your fist.
2.   If this procedure does not work, stand behind the victim and support his or her chest with one hand. With the heel of the other hand give 4 quick blows on the back between the victim's shoulder blades.

If You Are Alone and Choking:

1.   Place your fist on your stomach slightly above your navel and below your ribs. Place your other hand on top of it. Give yourself 4 quick, forceful upward abdominal thrusts.
2.   If this procedure does not work, press your stomach forcefully over a chair, table, sink, or railing.

FIRST-AID
TECHNIQUES TO LEARN
AND PRACTICE

Dressings, bandages, slings, and splints are an important part of first-aid care. It is a good idea to learn and practice their application before an emergency strikes. Knowing how to apply a dressing, bandage, or splint will enable you to do so calmly and expertly during a stressful situation.

DRESSINGS

A dressing, or compress, is a covering placed directly over a wound. Its purpose is to help control bleeding, absorb secretions from the wound, and prevent contamination by germs. Because the dressing is placed directly over the wound, it should be sterile. Sterile dressings such as gauze pads and bandages are individually wrapped and are available at most drugstores. If a sterile dressing is not available, a clean and freshly ironed handkerchief, pillowcase, sheet, or other cloth can be used. (Heat from an iron helps kill germs.) If time allows, a cloth boiled in water for 15 minutes and then dried will provide a sterile dressing. Adhesive tape and fluffy materials such as absorbent cotton should never be applied directly to the wound, as they can stick to the wound and are difficult to remove.

The dressing should be large enough to cover an area 1 inch beyond all edges of the wound, to prevent contamination of any part of the wound. To apply the dressing, hold it directly over the wound and lower it into place. *Do not* slide or drag the dressing over the skin, as this contaminates the dressing. Discard any dressing that has slipped out of place before it has been bandaged.

BANDAGES

A bandage is a piece of material that holds a dressing or splint in place. It can also be a wrap, such as an elastic bandage, that is applied directly to an injured area to help decrease bleeding or swelling or lend support to a joint or group of muscles.

To function properly, a bandage must be applied snugly *but not too tightly*. A bandage applied too tightly can cut off circulation and cause serious tissue damage. An elastic bandage, though very effective if applied properly, can be particularly dangerous because of the first-aider's tendency to stretch it too tightly. Remember that an injured area may swell, causing a snug bandage to become too tight.

When applying a bandage to the arm, hand, leg, or foot, leave the fingertips or toes exposed so that danger signals such as swelling, bluish or pale color, or coldness can be observed or felt. If any of these signs appear or if the victim complains of numbness or tingling, loosen the bandage immediately.

Types of Bandages

I. Rectangular Bandage

A rectangular bandage is used for simple cuts and abrasions and can be purchased at most drugstores. The rectangular bandage is a combination of both dressing and bandage. To prevent contamination, do not touch the gauze dressing while applying it to the wound.

Rectangular Bandage

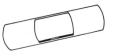

A rectangular bandage, a combination of both dressing and bandage, is used for simple cuts and abrasions.

II. Butterfly Bandage (tape) and Narrow Adhesive Strips

Butterfly bandages and narrow adhesive strips are thin pieces of tape that are used to hold the edges of a cut together, thus allowing the wound to heal. They are especially useful in treating small cuts and in cases in which a deep laceration has not occurred. When applying either tape, gently hold the edges of the cut together. (Either tape can be purchased at a drugstore. If the tapes are not available, ask your pharmacist where they might be purchased.)

Other Types of Bandages

The butterfly bandage *(left)* and the narrow adhesive strip *(right)* are thin pieces of tape that are used to hold the edges of a cut together.

III. Roller Gauze Bandage

The roller bandage comes in various widths and lengths and is usually made of gauze. It comes packaged in rolls and can be used on most parts of the body. If commercial roller bandages are not available, a bandage can be made from a clean strip of cloth. The most common uses of roller gauze are for circular, figure-of-eight, and fingertip bandages.

A **circular bandage** is the easiest to apply. It is used on areas that do not vary much in width, such as the wrist, toes, and fingers.

To apply a circular bandage:

1. Anchor the bandage by placing the end of the gauze at a slight angle over the affected part and making several circular turns to hold the end in place. Don't wrap the bandage too tightly, however.
2. Make additional circular turns by overlapping the preceding strip by approximately three-fourths of its width. Continue the bandage in the same direction until the dressing is completely covered.
3. To secure the bandage cut the gauze with scissors or a knife and apply adhesive tape or a safety pin to the bandage. Or tie a loop knot by extending the rolled gauze out about 8 inches away from the part being bandaged. Place your thumb or two fingers in the middle of the rolled-out gauze and pull that section of the gauze (from the fingers to the gauze roll) in the same direction as you did in applying the bandage. The remainder of the gauze and roll will be on the opposite side. Now, with the doubled gauze on one side and the single gauze on the other, tie a knot over the bandage. If scissors are available, cut off the unused gauze.

Circular Bandage

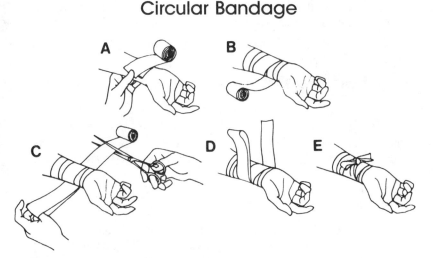

A. Anchor the bandage by placing the end of the gauze at a slight angle over the affected part and making several turns to hold the end in place.

B. Make additional turns by overlapping the preceding strip by approximately three-fourths of its width. Continue the bandage in the same direction until the dressing is completely covered.

C. To secure the bandage, cut the gauze and apply tape or a safety pin, *or* tie a loop knot by rolling the gauze out about 8 inches away from the part being bandaged. Place thumb in the middle of the rolled gauze and pull that section of the gauze (from your finger to the gauze roll) back under the wrist to the opposite side of the arm. If scissors are available, cut the gauze.

D. The doubled gauze is on one side and the single gauze is on the other.

E. Tie a knot over the bandage.

A **figure-of-eight bandage** is particularly useful for the ankle, wrist, and hand.

To apply a figure-of-eight bandage:

1. Anchor the bandage with one or two circular turns around the affected part. Don't wrap the bandage too tightly, however.

2. To make the figure-of-eight, bring the bandage diagonally across the top of the foot, around the ankle, down across the top of the foot, and under the arch. Continue these figure-of-eight turns, with each turn overlapping the preceding turn by about three-fourths of its width. Bandage until the foot (not toes), ankle, and lower part of the leg are covered.

3. Secure the bandage with tape, clips, or safety pins, or tie off as described in the section on the circular bandage.

Figure-of-Eight Bandage

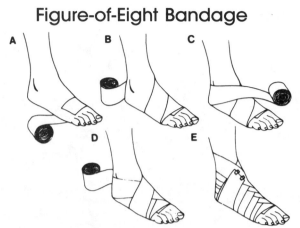

A. Anchor the bandage with 1 or 2 circular turns.
B. Bring the bandage diagonally across the top of the foot and around the heel and ankle.
C. Continue the bandage down across the top of the foot and under the arch.
D. Continue figure-of-eight turns, with each turn overlapping the preceding turn by about three-fourths of its width.
E. Bandage until the foot (not the toes), ankle, and lower leg are covered. Secure the bandage with tape or clips.

The **fingertip bandage** is particularly useful when the fingertip itself is injured.

To apply a fingertip bandage:

1. Anchor the bandage at the base of the finger with a few circular turns. Don't wrap the bandage too tightly, however.
2. With your index finger of one hand, hold the bandage down at the base where it is anchored. Bring the roll of bandage up the front of the finger you are bandaging, over the fingertip, and down the back side to the base of the finger.
3. Now, with your thumb, hold down the bandage at the base and repeat the back-and-forth process of bandaging over the fingertip as described. Repeat bandaging until several layers cover the finger.
4. Next, starting at the base of the finger, make circular turns up the finger and back to the base to hold the bandage in place.
5. To secure the bandage, apply a piece of tape approximately 6 inches long up the side of the finger, across the tip, and down the other side of the finger. Or tie off as described in the section on the circular bandage.

Fingertip Bandage

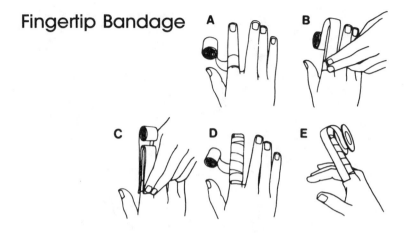

A. Anchor the bandage at the base of the finger with several circular turns.
B. Hold the bandage down at the base where it is anchored. Bring the bandage up the front of the finger, over the fingertip, and down the back side to the base of the finger.
C. Hold down the bandage at the base with the thumb. Repeat the back-and-forth bandaging process over the fingertip until several layers cover the finger.
D. To hold the bandage in place, start at the base of the finger and make circular turns up the finger and back to the base.
E. To secure the bandage, apply a piece of tape about 6 inches long up the side of the finger, across the tip, and down the other side of the finger.

IV. Triangular Bandage

The triangular bandage has many uses in an emergency. It can serve as a covering for a large area such as the scalp or as a sling for a broken bone, or it can be folded into a rectangular scarf and used as a circular or figure-of-eight bandage. A triangular bandage is usually made of muslin, but other material can be used. It can be

Triangular Bandage

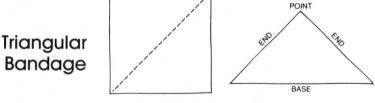

A triangular bandage can be used as a sling, as a head bandage, or as a (rectangular) figure-of-eight bandage. (Refer to illustrations on the following pages.)

easily made at home. To make a triangular bandage, cut a piece of cloth 36 to 40 inches square. Next cut the fabric diagonally from corner to corner. Now you have two triangular bandages.

To make a sling:

1. Place one *end* of the bandage over the uninjured shoulder so that the *base* and other *end* of the triangle hang down over the chest. Place the *point* under the elbow of the injured arm.
2. Elevate the hand about 4 inches above the level of the elbow.
3. Lift the lower end of the bandage up over the other shoulder and tie the two ends together at the side of the neck.
4. Fold the point forward and pin it to the outside of the sling.
5. *Do not* cover the fingers with the sling.

Sling

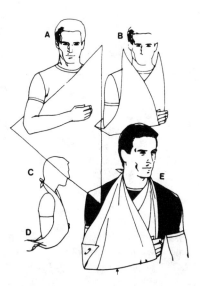

A. Place one *end* of the bandage over the uninjured shoulder. The *base* and other *end* of the triangle hang down over the chest. Place the *point* under the elbow of the injured arm.
B. Elevate the hand about 4 inches above the level of the elbow. Lift the lower end of the bandage up over the other shoulder and tie the two ends together at the *side* of the neck.
C. Tie at the neck.
D. Fold the point forward and pin it to the outside of the sling.
E. Completed sling, with the point folded and pinned to the outside of the sling. Leave the fingers exposed.

To make a head bandage:

1.   Place the center of the base of the triangle across the forehead so that it lies just above the eyes. The point of the bandage should lie down the back of the head.
2.   Bring both ends above the ears and around to the back of the head. Just below the lump at the back of the head, cross the two ends over each other snugly and continue to bring the ends back around to the center of the forehead.
3.   Tie the ends in a knot.
4.   Tuck the point hanging down the back of the head into the fold where the bandage crosses in the back.

Head Bandage

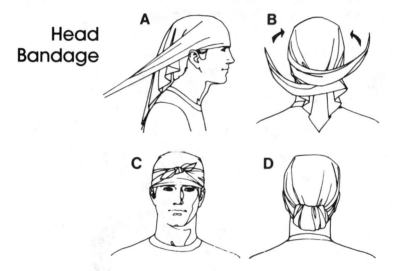

A. Place the center of the triangle base across the forehead so that it lies just above the eyes, with the point of the bandage down the back of the head. Bring the ends above the ears and around to the back of the head.
B. Cross the two ends snugly over each other just below the lump at the back of the head. Bring the ends back around to the center of the forehead.
C. Tie the ends in a knot.
D. Tuck the point in the fold where the bandage crosses.

The triangular bandage can be folded as a *scarf* or *necktie bandage* and then used as a circular or figure-of-eight bandage. To make a cravat (scarf or necktie) bandage:

1. Fold the point of the bandage over to the middle of the base.
2. Continue to fold the bandage lengthwise along the middle until the bandage is the desired width.

Cravat (Scarf or Necktie) Bandage

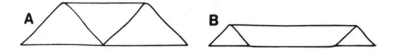

A. Fold the point of the triangle bandage to the middle of the base.
B. Continue folding lengthwise along the middle until the bandage is the desired width.

SPLINTS

Splints are used to keep an injured part from moving. They ease pain and help prevent shock.

Objects that can be used for splinting include boards, straight sticks, brooms, pieces of corrugated cardboard bent to form a three-sided box, rolled newspapers or magazines, pillows, rolled blankets, oars, or umbrellas. The splint should extend above and below the injured area to immobilize it.

Padding such as cloth, towels, or blankets should be placed between the splint and the skin of the injured part.

Splints can be tied in place with neckties, strips of cloth torn from shirts, handkerchiefs, belts, string, rope, or other suitable material.

Do not tie the splint so tightly that the ties interfere with circulation. Swelling or bluish discoloration in the fingers or toes may indicate that the ties are too tight and need to be loosened. Also loosen splint ties if the victim experiences numbness or tingling, or if he or she cannot move the fingers or toes. Check the wrist or ankle for a pulse and loosen the ties if no pulse can be felt.

To splint specific broken bones, see Broken Bones and Spinal Injuries in Part II.

PART II

ALPHABETICAL LISTING OF INJURIES AND ILLNESSES

ABDOMINAL PAIN

There are hundreds of causes of abdominal pain. Some are serious and require immediate medical care. If symptoms are severe or persist, regardless of whether they fall into any of the following categories, seek medical attention promptly. A victim of severe abdominal pain should never be given an enema, a laxative, medication, food, or liquids (including water) without a doctor's advice, since doing so may aggravate the problem or cause a complication.

Abdomen

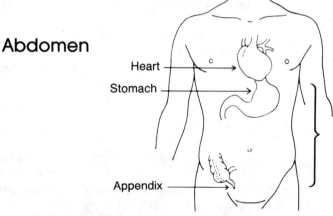

The *abdomen* is the part of the body located between the diaphragm (a muscle) and the pelvis. It includes such organs as the liver, stomach, pancreas, gallbladder, intestines, and appendix. The heart lies above the abdomen and is separated from it by the diaphragm.

APPENDICITIS

Appendicitis is a surgical emergency. It results when the appendix becomes inflamed and infected. Immediate surgical removal of the appendix is necessary.

Symptoms   Any or all of the following may be present:

1. Pain, usually beginning intermittently in a generalized area around the navel and later moving to the lower right part of the abdomen, where it may become constant. Pain is not always severe.
2. Fever.
3. Nausea and vomiting.
4. Loss of appetite.
5. Usually, lack of bowel movements. But diarrhea may occur sporadically.
6. Tenderness in the abdomen, especially in the right lower quarter when touched, or when the area is pressed, then released rapidly.

NOTE: *Appendicitis in children does not follow the same pattern that occurs in adults.* Children may exhibit only a few symptoms, such as lack of appetite and a tender abdomen.

Immediate Treatment
1. *Do not* give the victim laxatives, enemas, medication, food, or liquids (including water).
2. Seek medical attention promptly, preferably at the nearest hospital emergency room. Delay can be serious. Perforation (rupture) of the appendix can occur.

BOWEL OBSTRUCTION

A bowel obstruction is a partial or complete blockage in the bowel that causes interference in the passage of waste material through the bowel. This blockage may be caused by adhesions (scar formation) following surgery, an abscess, tumors, or a "kink" or twist (malrotation) in the bowel. Bowel obstruction is usually a surgical emergency.

Symptoms   Any or all of the following may be present:

1. Severe, cramplike pain in the abdomen that subsides, then repeats and becomes increasingly severe.
2. Nausea and vomiting.
3. Expansion of the abdomen, which then becomes firmer than normal.

4. Diarrhea, constipation, or any change in bowel habits.
5. Any one or all of the above may be present.

Immediate
Treatment

Do not give the victim laxatives, enemas, medication, food, or liquids (including water). Seek medical attention promptly, even with the slightest suspicion of bowel obstruction. Delay can cause gangrene and loss of part of the bowel.

CRAMPS, MENSTRUAL

Cramping pains in the mid-lower abdomen are common during menstruation. They usually occur at the beginning of the period and may last for several days.

What to Do

1. If there is no doubt that the pain is caused by menstrual cramps, a mild pain reliever, such as aspirin, ibuprofen, or acetaminophen, or a product made specifically for menstrual cramps, is often helpful.
2. Pain, however, can be severe and incapacitating. If it persists or is greater than usual, medical attention is needed to rule out a more serious problem.

ECTOPIC PREGNANCY

An ectopic pregnancy is a pregnancy that develops outside of the uterus, usually in the Fallopian tubes, and is a serious surgical emergency. *It is one of the leading causes of maternal death.* As the embryo grows, it becomes too large for the narrow Fallopian tube. Rupture of the tube usually occurs during the second or third month of pregnancy. A ruptured Fallopian tube is a surgical emergency because excessive internal bleeding into the abdomen can occur, leading to shock or death.

Symptoms

Any or all of the following may be present:

1. Usually, the menstrual period is late, prolonged, or missed.
2. Pain occurs on one side of the lower abdomen, but it may not be severe until the Fallopian tube ruptures.

3. Vaginal bleeding may occur prior to, or with, abdominal pain.
4. The victim may become pale and perspire.
5. Pulse may be rapid.
6. Pain may also be present in the shoulder area.

Immediate
Treatment

1. *Do not* give the victim laxatives, enemas, medication, food, or liquids (including water).
2. Seek medical attention promptly. Surgery most likely will be necessary.

GALLBLADDER INFLAMMATION

Sudden inflammation of the gallbladder is called cholecystitis. It usually occurs when gallstones are present, but can occur in their absence. The condition occurs most often among 30- to 50-year-olds.

Symptoms   Any or all of the following may be present:

1. Upper abdominal discomfort or pain that may subside, changing to severe pain in the upper right abdomen.
2. Radiation of pain to the back, below the right shoulder blade.
3. Loss of appetite.
4. Slight fever.
5. Nausea and vomiting.

Immediate
Treatment

Seek medical attention promptly, preferably at the nearest hospital emergency room.

KIDNEY STONE PAIN

The problem occurs when a kidney stone moves from the kidney down the ureter, irritating the ureter wall and causing spasms. The stone can obstruct urine flow and is a medical emergency.

Symptoms   Any or all of the following may be present:

1. Excruciating pain in the side or back.
2. Radiation of pain to the groin.
3. Sweating.
4. Facial pallor.
5. Nausea and occasional vomiting.

Immediate   Seek medical attention promptly, preferably at the
Treatment   nearest hospital emergency room.

PANCREATITIS

Sudden inflammation of the pancreas is called acute pancreatitis. It
can occur with or follow gallbladder disease (stones) in the middle-
aged and elderly. In younger individuals, the condition can be
brought on by drinking alcoholic beverages.

Symptoms   Any or all of the following may be present:

1. Sudden onset of severe, unrelenting pain in the middle of the
    upper abdomen. Pain may also be present in the middle of the
    lower back.
2. Increased pain, aggravated by any movement or from pressure
    placed on the abdomen.
3. Facial pallor.
4. Sweating.
5. Rapid pulse.
6. Nausea and vomiting.

Immediate   Seek medical attention promptly, preferably at the
Treatment   nearest hospital emergency room.

ABDOMINAL PAIN IN INFANTS AND CHILDREN

Abdominal pain in infants can be *very* serious and needs medical
attention. An infant usually indicates abdominal pain by crying
loudly, bending the legs, and drawing the knees toward the chest.
    Serious problems that can occur in infancy and that require
prompt medical attention are discussed briefly below.

Twist in the Bowel (Malrotation):

Usually occurs between 1 and 12 months. Symptoms may include
vomiting (vomit may show greenish-brown bile) and abdominal dis-
tention, in which the stomach swells and is hard to the touch. There
may also be streaks of blood in the infant's stool.

Strangulated (Incarcerated) Hernia:

A bent and trapped loop of bowel. There may be a mass (hard lump) you can feel in the scrotum or inguinal (groin or lower abdomen) area. It can occur at any age. Symptoms include irritability and vomiting.

Pyloric Stenosis:

Narrowing of the outlet of the stomach resulting in **projectile vomiting** (food that is expelled with force by the infant, usually right after feeding). Usually occurs in male infants, 3 to 6 weeks of age.

Intussusception:

A part of the bowel that becomes engulfed in a portion of bowel next to it in a telescoping fashion. Usually occurs in infants, 8 to 18 months old. Abdominal pain may occur suddenly, then subside, then recur without warning. Infant may also have a red, jellylike stool.

Immediate Treatment

1. For any of these conditions, seek medical attention at once, preferably at the nearest hospital emergency room.
2. *Do not* give the infant laxatives, enemas, medication, food, or liquids (including water).

Abdominal pain in children is not unusual. Almost all children experience a stomachache at some time. A stomachache is usually not serious if it lasts less than an hour and there are no other symptoms such as fever, cough, headache, vomiting, or diarrhea.

What to Do

1. Whenever in doubt about symptoms, seek medical advice, *especially* if the symptoms increase in frequency and severity.
2. *Do not* give the child laxatives, enemas, medication, food, or liquids (including water).

See Also: Appendicitis, p. 53; Diarrhea, p. 144; Food Poisoning, p. 183; Miscarriage, p. 207; Pregnancy, Danger Signs, p. 221; Vomiting, p. 255; Wounds (abdominal), p. 257.

ALTITUDE SICKNESS

The illness is caused by the lack of oxygen in the air and decreased barometric pressure at high altitudes (above 10,000 feet).

Symptoms   Any or all of the following may be present:

1. Headache.
2. Extreme tiredness.
3. Lightheadedness.
4. Feeling of not being able to catch one's breath. The victim may try to breathe in more air, causing hyperventilation.
5. Pain in the chest, tightness in the throat.
6. Restlessness, inability to sleep.
7. Nausea and vomiting.
8. Fainting.
9. Hallucinations.
10. Panic.

ABCs

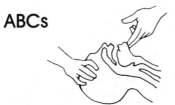

With all serious injuries, check and maintain an open airway. Restore breathing (p. 20) and circulation (p. 22), if necessary.

Immediate Treatment

1. Maintain an open airway. Restore breathing and circulation if necessary.
2. Keep the victim quiet, to conserve oxygen and energy. Have the victim breathe air from an auxiliary oxygen source, if available.
3. If the victim is breathing on his or her own, *do not* breathe more air, by mouth-to-mouth resuscitation, into the victim's lungs.

4. Keep the victim at rest until he or she can catch his or her breath. It is *very* important for you and others to remain calm, so that the victim will remain calm.

5. The victim may need to return to a lower altitude.

6. *Do not* send the victim off alone. Stay with him or her.

7. Suggest that the victim seek medical treatment.

ASTHMA

Asthma is a condition resulting from a gradual or sudden narrowing of the airway bronchial tubes in the lungs, causing difficulty in breathing. Breathing may be especially difficult when exhaling. Often, but not always, an attack results from exposure to something to which the victim is allergic. However, infections (bronchitis), exercise, cold weather, inhaled irritants in the air, or emotional factors can also lead to an attack.

Symptoms   Any or all of the following may be present:

1. Difficulty in exhaling. A wheezing or whistling sound is heard as air is forced out through narrow airways.
2. Nervousness, tenseness, fright.
3. Coughing.
4. Possible perspiration on forehead.
5. Choking sensation.
6. Possible vomiting.
7. Possible slight fever.
8. Bluish tinge to the skin in severe attacks, due to the lack of adequate oxygen intake.
9. The victim always tries to sit upright because doing so makes it easier for him or her to breathe.

What to Do   If this is the first episode of suspected but undiagnosed asthma, seek medical attention. Report all details of the attack. If a doctor cannot be reached, take the victim to the nearest hospital emergency room. Comfort and reassure the victim, particularly a child who may be frightened by the experience, since emotional stress may make the condition worse. Keep the victim in a sitting position. Don't force the victim to lie down.

If attacks have occurred before, give the victim prescribed medications according to the instructions on the container. Do not give the victim anything else without a physician's advice. Report the attack to the victim's physician.

Danger Signals   If symptoms continue and one or more of the following happens:

1. Failure to improve with medication.
2. Difficulty inhaling or inability to exhale; breathing becomes barely audible.
3. Inability to cough.
4. Increased bluish tinge to skin.
5. Increased pulse rate, to more than 120 beats per minute.
6. Increased anxiety.

WARNING: If the victim tries to pull up the shoulders and chin to expand the chest to get air, *seek medical attention at once.* Call paramedics or go to the nearest hospital emergency room. This is a dire medical emergency. The victim may be near respiratory failure and could collapse.

BITES AND STINGS

ANIMAL BITES

Animal bites can result in serious infections as well as in tissue damage. Cat scratches can be particularly serious as well, as they may cause cat-scratch fever (a glandular infection). Many animals including bats, skunks, squirrels, raccoons, foxes, rats, cats, and dogs can transmit rabies as well as tetanus.

What to Do
1. Clean the wound thoroughly with soap and running water for 5 minutes or more to wash out contaminating organisms.
2. Put a sterile bandage or clean cloth over the wound.
3. Seek medical attention promptly, particularly for a bite on the face, neck, or hands, which frequently can develop into a serious infection.
4. If some skin tissue, such as a part of an ear or a nose, is bitten off, bring it to the hospital with the victim.

NOTE: *It is very important to catch and confine any animal that has bitten someone, so that it can be observed and evaluated for rabies. Capture the animal alive if possible. If it is absolutely necessary to kill the animal, try to avoid damage to the head. Save the body for examination by health department officials. If the animal cannot be captured or killed, try to remember its physical characteristics and its actions, so that the animal can be identified.*
Notify the police and local health department.

HUMAN BITES

Any human bite that breaks the skin needs immediate medical treatment. Human bites can lead to very serious infections from oral bacteria or viruses that may contaminate the wound. A bite on the hand, in particular, can cause loss of the use of the fingers and of the hand.

Immediate
Treatment

1. Clean the wound thoroughly with soap and running water for 5 minutes or more to irrigate the wound. This washes out any contaminating organisms.
2. *Do not* put medication, antiseptics, or home remedies on the wound.
3. Put a sterile bandage or clean cloth over the wound.
4. Seek medical attention promptly. *Don't wait.*

INSECT STINGS

Though most stings cause only local reactions (redness, swelling), some insect stings can be life-threatening if the victim is allergic to the insect's venom. (See Allergic Reactions to Insect Stings, following this section.)

Insect stings cause more deaths per year than snakebites. The most common stinging insects are honeybees, hornets, wasps, yellow jackets, bumblebees, and fire ants.

Symptoms   Any or all of the following may be present:

1. Pain.
2. Local swelling.
3. Redness.
4. Itching.
5. Burning.

Symptoms occur at the bite area and may last 48 to 72 hours.

What to Do

1. When a honeybee stings, it usually leaves behind its stinger. Carefully remove the stinger by gently scraping the skin with a knife blade, card edge, or fingernail. *Do not* squeeze with tweezers, as this may result in more venom

entering the body, through the compression of the stinger sac.

2. Wash the area with soap and water.
3. Place ice wrapped in cloth or cold compresses on the sting area to decrease the absorption and spread of the venom.
4. Soothing lotions, such as calamine, or a paste of baking soda and a little water are often helpful in relieving discomfort.
5. An antihistamine may ease the symptoms.

Allergic Reactions to Insect Stings

An allergic reaction to insect stings can be life-threatening and can occur from one or more bites or stings. Allergic reactions often occur if the victim has been bitten or stung previously.

Anaphylactic shock is a generalized total body allergic reaction that can occur from such stings. (See Shock from an Allergic Reaction, p. 234.)

Symptoms   Any or all of the following may be present:

1. Severe swelling in other parts of the body such as the eyes, lips, and tongue, as well as at the bite site.
2. Hives or hivelike rash on the body.
3. Coughing or wheezing.
4. Severe itching.
5. Difficulty in breathing.
6. Stomach cramps.
7. Nausea and vomiting.
8. Anxiety.
9. Weakness.
10. Dizziness.
11. Possible bluish tinge to the skin.
12. Collapse.
13. Possible unconsciousness.

Immediate Treatment   If an emergency kit for insect stings is *not* available:

1. Maintain an open airway. Restore breathing and circulation, if necessary.

INJURIES AND ILLNESSES

2. If stung by a honeybee, carefully remove the stinger by gently scraping with a knife blade, card edge, or fingernail.

Do not squeeze the stinger with tweezers, as this may result in more venom entering the body.

3. If the victim experiences the symptoms listed that suggest a severe allergic reaction *and* the victim is known to have had previous severe reactions to insect stings, the use of a tourniquet may be necessary. Although not all experts agree on this method, many allergists recommend the use of a tourniquet to prevent severe reactions where the victim's life is at stake. Emergency insect sting kits available only by prescription contain a tourniquet for such cases. A tourniquet helps to slow the flow of blood and absorption of the venom throughout the body.

The tourniquet is used only if the sting has just occurred and is on the arm or leg. A rubber tourniquet works best, but a strip of cloth or cord may be used.

Tie the tourniquet 2 to 4 inches above the sting, between the sting and the body. *Do not* tie so tightly that the victim's arterial circulation is cut off completely. *Be sure* you can find a pulse below the tourniquet. Loosen the tourniquet about every 5 minutes until medical assistance is obtained.

4. If the victim experiences severe symptoms of an allergic reaction but has no known previous history of severe reactions to insect stings and the sting has just occurred on the arm or leg, apply a light constricting band, such as an elastic watchband, belt, or

Light Tourniquet

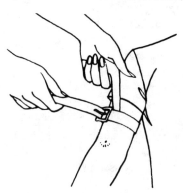

A light constricting band is used for *severe* reactions to insect stings and for rattlesnake, copperhead, and cottonmouth (not coral) snakebites. Place the band 2 to 4 inches above the bite, between the bite and the body. *Do not* cut off arterial circulation. You should be able to slip your finger under the band.

tie, 2 to 4 inches above the sting, between the sting and the body. The band *should not* be so tight that it cuts off arterial circulation. You should feel a pulse *below* the band. You should be able to slip your finger under the band. *Do not* remove the band until medical assistance is obtained.

5. Seek medical attention promptly, preferably at the nearest hospital emergency room.

Continued Care

1. Place cold compresses on the sting area to stop absorption and spread of the injected venom.
2. Keep victim lying down unless he or she is short of breath; then let victim sit up slowly.
3. Keep the victim comfortable and quiet.

If an emergency kit for insect stings is available:

Immediate Treatment

1. Maintain an open airway. Restore breathing and circulation, if necessary.
2. Remove the stinger if stung by a honeybee. Carefully remove the stinger by gently scraping the skin with a knife blade, card edge, or fingernail. *Do not* squeeze the stinger with tweezers, as this may result in more venom entering the body.
3. If the victim is unable to administer an injection of adrenaline, follow instructions in the emergency kit.
4. Seek medical attention promptly, preferably at the nearest hospital emergency room, or call paramedics if available.

Continued Care

See Continued Care above.

MULTIPLE STINGS (TOXIC REACTION)

Symptoms   Any or all of the following may be present:

1. Rapid onset of swelling.
2. Headache.
3. Muscle cramps.
4. Fever.
5. Drowsiness.
6. Unconsciousness.

INJURIES AND ILLNESSES

What to Do   1.   Remove stingers if the victim was stung by honeybees. (See Allergic Reactions to Insect Stings—Immediate Treatment, p. 65.)
2.   Wash the sting sites with soap and water.
3.   Place ice wrapped in cloth or cold compresses on sting sites.
4.   Soothing lotions, such as calamine or a paste of baking soda and a little water, are often helpful in relieving discomfort.
5.   Seek medical attention, as other medication may be needed.

SPIDER BITES

Black Widow Spider Bites

Black widow spider bites are particularly harmful to very young children, the elderly, and the chronically ill.

Black Widow Spider

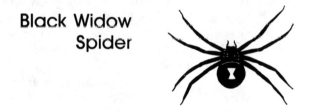

The *black widow spider* has a shiny black body. Its unique feature is a red hourglass marking on the underside of its body.

Symptoms   Any or all of the following may be present:

1.   Slight redness and swelling around the bite.
2.   Sharp pain around the bite.
3.   Profuse sweating.
4.   Nausea and possible vomiting.
5.   Stomach cramps or hard, rigid abdomen.
6.   Possible muscle cramps in other parts of the body.
7.   Tightness in the chest and difficulty in breathing and talking.

Immediate   1.   Maintain an open airway and restore breathing, if necessary.
Treatment

ABCs

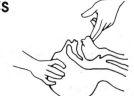

With all serious injuries, check and maintain an open *airway*. Restore *breathing* (p. 20) and *circulation* (p. 22), if necessary.

2. Keep the bitten area lower than the victim's heart.
3. Place ice wrapped in cloth or cold compresses on the bitten area.
4. Seek medical attention promptly, preferably at the nearest hospital emergency room. If possible, take the spider with you.

Continued Care

1. Keep the victim quiet.
2. Watch for signs of shock and treat if necessary. (See Shock, p. 234.)

Brown Recluse Spider (Fiddleback Spider) Bites

Brown recluse spider bites are particularly harmful to very young children. The spider's bite causes severe, deep, irreversible tissue damage around the bite area. Immediate medical attention is required.

Brown Recluse Spider

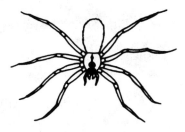

The *brown recluse spider* (also called the fiddleback or violin spider) is characterized by a dark brown violin-shaped marking on the top front portion of its body.

Symptoms   Any or all of the following may be present:

1. The victim feels a stinging sensation at the time of the bite.
2. Redness occurs, which later disappears as a blister forms.
3. If the bite is not treated promptly, pain becomes more severe during the following 8 hours.
4. Over the next 48 hours, chills, fever, nausea, vomiting, joint pains, and possible rash appear.
5. Destruction of tissue forms an open ulcer.

Immediate   See Immediate Treatment under Black Widow Spi-
Treatment   der Bites, pp. 68–69.

Continued   See Continued Care under Black Widow Spider
Care   Bites, p. 69.

Tarantula Bites

Tarantula bites are not usually as serious as those of the black widow spider or the brown recluse spider.

Tarantula

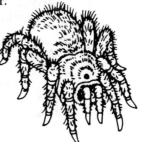

The *tarantula* is a large spider with a very hairy body and legs.

Symptoms   Either or both symptoms may be present:

1. Pain is usually not severe at the time of the bite.
2. A severe, painful wound may develop later.

What to Do   1. Wash the area with soap and water.
             2. Place ice wrapped in cloth or cold compresses on the bite area.
             3. Soothing lotions such as calamine may be helpful in relieving discomfort.

4. If a severe reaction occurs, see Immediate Treatment and Continued Care under Black Widow Spider Bites, pp. 68–69.
5. Seek medical attention.

MARINE LIFE STINGS

Stings from certain types of marine life are poisonous. Two of the most common offenders are the Portuguese man-of-war and the jellyfish.

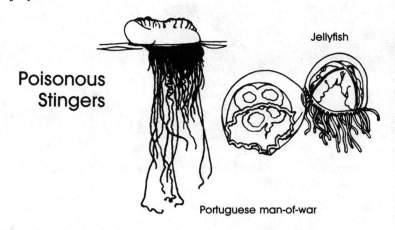

Poisonous
Stingers

Jellyfish

Portuguese man-of-war

Stings from the Portuguese man-of-war and the jellyfish are poisonous.

Symptoms   Any or all of the following may be present:

1. Intense burning pain.
2. Reddening of the skin.
3. Skin rash.
4. Muscle cramps.
5. Nausea and vomiting.
6. Difficulty in breathing.
7. Possible shock, due to severe allergic reaction.

What to Do
1. If stung by a Portuguese man-of-war, wrap cloth around your hands (or use tweezers, pliers, or forceps) and then carefully remove any attached tentacles. *An unattached tentacle can still sting.*
2. Wash the area with rubbing alcohol or vinegar. (Doing so may cause a stinging sensation.)

3. Watch for signs of shock and treat if necessary. (See Shock, pp. 234–237.)
4. Seek medical attention.

SCORPION STINGS

Some species of scorpions are more poisonous than others. Scorpion stings are particularly harmful to very young children.

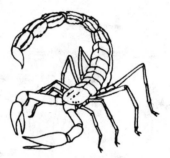

Scorpion

The *scorpion* looks like a small lobster. It has a set of pincers and a stinger located in the tail, which arches over its back.

Symptoms   Any or all of the following may be present:

1. Severe burning pain at the site of the sting.
2. Nausea and vomiting.
3. Stomach pain.
4. Numbness and tingling in the affected area.
5. Possible spasm of jaw muscles, making opening of the mouth difficult.
6. Twitching and spasm of affected muscles.
7. Shock. (See Shock, pp. 234–237.)
8. Convulsions.
9. Possible coma.

Immediate   1. Maintain an open airway. Restore breathing
Treatment   and circulation, if necessary.
              2. Keep the bitten area lower than the victim's heart.

ABCs

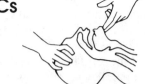

With all serious injuries, check and maintain an open *airway*. Restore *breathing* (p. 20) and *circulation* (p. 22), if necessary.

3. Place ice wrapped in cloth or cold compresses on the bitten area.
4. Seek medical attention promptly, preferably at the nearest hospital emergency room.

Continued Care

1. Keep the victim quiet.
2. Watch for signs of shock and treat if necessary. (See Shock, pp. 234–237.)

SNAKEBITES

When you are bitten by a snake, it is important to know whether or not it is poisonous. Poisonous snakes in the United States include the **rattlesnake, cottonmouth (water moccasin), copperhead, and coral snake.** Rattlesnakes can be found all over the country. Cottonmouth and copperhead snakes are found primarily in the southeast and south-central parts of the United States. Coral snakes are found primarily in the southeast.

Rattlesnake

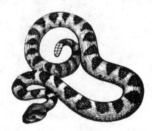

The *rattlesnake* has deep poison pits located between the nostrils and the eyes. It has slitlike eyes and two long fangs. A unique feature of the rattlesnake is the set of rattles at the end of the tail.

The rattlesnake, cottonmouth, and copperhead have a triangular-shaped head and are pit vipers, recognized by deep pits (poison sacs) located between the nostrils and the eyes. They also have slitlike eyes rather than the rounded eyes of the nonpoisonous snakes (with the exception of the coral snake). These snakes also have long fangs that leave distinctive marks followed by a row of tooth marks. Rattlesnakes get their name from a set of rattles at the end of their tail. Cottonmouths have white coloring inside their mouths.

Cottonmouth

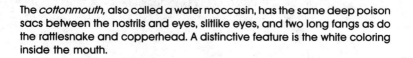

The *cottonmouth,* also called a water moccasin, has the same deep poison sacs between the nostrils and eyes, slitlike eyes, and two long fangs as do the rattlesnake and copperhead. A distinctive feature is the white coloring inside the mouth.

The coral snake is a member of the cobra family. It has red, yellow, and black rings. The yellow rings are narrow and *always* separate the red rings from the black. A rhyme to remember that identifies the coral snake is "Red on yellow will kill a fellow, red on black won't hurt Jack." The coral snake is smaller than the pit vipers, has rounded eyes like nonpoisonous snakes, and *always* has a black nose. Its venom is highly toxic to humans.

Coral Snake

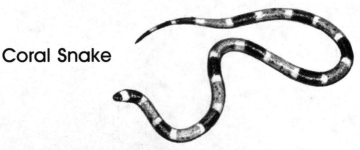

Unlike the rattlesnake, copperhead, and cottonmouth, the *coral snake* has rounded eyes. The coral snake also has fangs. Its markings consist of yellow, red, and black rings, with the narrow yellow rings *always* separating the red rings from the black. The coral snake *always* has a black nose.

Nonpoisonous snakes have rounded eyes. They do not have pits between their eyes and nostrils and do not have fangs.

Triangular-Shaped Head of a Poisonous Snake

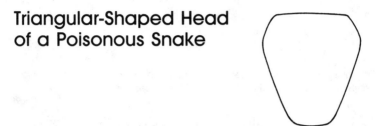

The rattlesnake, copperhead, and cottonmouth all have a triangular-shaped head.

Try to capture and kill the snake, if possible without deforming its head, and take it with you to the medical facility. If this is impossible, remember the characteristics of the snake.

Characteristics of a Poisonous Snake

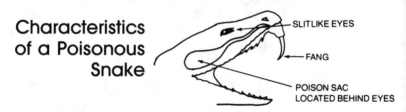

SLITLIKE EYES

FANG

POISON SAC LOCATED BEHIND EYES

The rattlesnake, copperhead, and cottonmouth all share these characteristics.

If Bitten by a Rattlesnake, Cottonmouth, or Copperhead:

Symptoms   Any or all of the following may be present:

1. Severe pain.
2. Rapid swelling.
3. Discoloration of the skin around the bite.
4. Weakness.
5. Nausea and vomiting.
6. Difficulty in breathing.
7. Blurring vision.
8. Convulsions.
9. Shock.

INJURIES AND ILLNESSES

ABCs

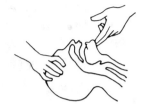

With all serious injuries, check and maintain an open *airway*. Restore *breathing* (p. 20) and *circulation* (p. 22), if necessary.

Immediate Treatment

1. Maintain an open airway. Restore breathing and circulation if necessary.
2. Keep the victim quiet to slow circulation. Doing so will help stop the spread of the venom.
3. If the victim was bitten on the arm or leg, place a light constricting band such as a belt or elastic watchband 2 to 4 inches above the bite, between the bite and the body. The band should not be so tight that it cuts off arterial circulation. You should feel a pulse *below* the band.

Light Tourniquet

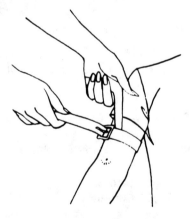

A light constricting band is used for *severe* reactions to insect stings (see Insect Stings, Anaphylactic Shock in text) and for rattlesnake, copperhead, and cottonmouth (not coral) snakebites. A light tourniquet of this sort restricts the blood flow and absorption of venom in the body. Place the band 2 to 4 inches above the bite, between the bite and the body. *Do not* cut off arterial circulation. You should be able to slip your finger under the band, although with some resistance.

You should be able to slip your finger under the band, although with some resistance. The wound should ooze.

4. If the area around the band should begin to swell, remove the band and place it 2 to 4 inches above the first site.

5. *Do not* remove the band or bands until medical assistance is obtained.

6. Wash the bite area thoroughly with soap and water.

7. Immobilize a bitten arm or leg with a splint or other suitable device.

8. *If a snakebite kit is available,* use the blade provided in the kit; otherwise, sterilize a knife blade over a flame. This must be done immediately after the victim has been bitten. Carefully make a ⅛- to ¼-inch-deep cut through each fang mark in the direction of the *length* of the arm or leg. The cut should not be more than ½ inch long.

To Remove Venom

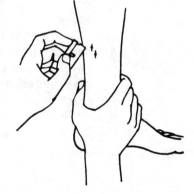

If bitten by a copperhead, cottonmouth, or rattlesnake (not coral snake), immediately make a ⅛- to ¼-inch-deep cut with a sterile blade through each fang mark in the direction of the length of the arm or leg.

Do not make cross-mark cuts. Be very careful not to cut any deeper than the skin, as muscle, nerve, or tendon damage may occur, particularly on the wrist, hand, or foot.

9. If suction cups are available, place them over victim's wound and draw out body fluids containing venom; otherwise use your mouth if it is free of cuts and sores.

Do not swallow the venom. Spit it out. Continue suction for 30 minutes or more. If the mouth method is used, rinse the mouth when finished.

WARNING: *Never* use cold or ice compresses on the wound as this may result in extensive tissue damage.

Continued Care

1. Cover the wound with a sterile or clean bandage.
2. Keep the victim quiet, calm, and reassured.
3. Treat the victim for shock. (See Shock, pp. 235–237.)
4. *Do not* let the victim walk unless absolutely necessary and, if so, then slowly.
5. The victim may have small sips of water if desired and if he or she has no difficulty swallowing. *Do not* give water if the victim is nauseated, vomiting, having convulsions, or unconscious.
6. *Do not* give the victim alcoholic beverages.
7. Seek medical attention promptly, preferably at the nearest hospital emergency room. If possible, have someone telephone ahead to tell of the poisonous snakebite and type of snake so that antivenom serum can be readied.

If Bitten by a Coral Snake:

Symptoms

Some symptoms may not occur immediately. Any or all of the following may be present:

1. Slight pain and swelling at the site of the bite.
2. Blurred vision.
3. Drooping eyelids.
4. Difficulty in speaking.
5. Heavy drooling.
6. Drowsiness.
7. Heavy sweating.
8. Nausea and vomiting.
9. Difficulty in breathing.
10. Paralysis.
11. Shock. (See Shock, pp. 234–237.)

Immediate Treatment

1. Quickly wash the affected area.
2. Immobilize a bitten arm or leg with a splint or other suitable device. (See Splinting and Other Procedures, pp. 95–107.)
3. Keep the victim quiet.
4. Seek medical assistance promptly, preferably at the nearest hospital emergency room. If possible, have someone call ahead to notify the hospital of the poisonous snakebite and type of snake so that antivenom serum can be ready.
5. *Do not* tie off the bite area.
6. *Do not* apply cold or ice compresses.
7. *Do not* give the victim food or alcoholic beverages.

If Bitten by a Nonpoisonous Snake:

What to Do

1. Keep the affected area below the level of the victim's heart.
2. Clean the area thoroughly with soap and water.
3. Put a bandage or clean cloth over the wound.
4. Seek medical attention, as medication or a tetanus shot may be necessary.

See Also: Rashes (Bites and Stings), p. 226; Shock (Shock from an Allergic Reaction to Insect Stings), p. 234; Unconsciousness, p. 251.

INJURIES AND ILLNESSES

BLEEDING

Blood may flow from a vein or an artery or both. Venous bleeding is darker red in color and flows steadily. Arterial bleeding is bright red in color and usually spurts from the wound. Arterial bleeding is more critical because blood is being pumped out at a faster rate, leading to greater blood loss.*

ABCs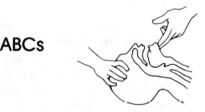

With all serious injuries, check and maintain an open airway. Restore breathing (p. 20) and circulation (p. 22), if necessary.

EXTERNAL BLEEDING

Immediate Treatment

I. Direct Pressure

Direct pressure is the preferred treatment in bleeding injuries and, though it may cause some pain, constant pressure is usually all that is necessary to stop the bleeding.

*NOTE: There is concern among those who provide first aid—even on a onetime basis—that AIDS may be contracted from a victim's body fluids. It is *extremely unlikely* that you—as a first-aider providing emergency care—will contract AIDS from a victim who is bleeding or from the saliva of a victim who may require mouth-to-mouth resuscitation or CPR.

AIDS is present in individuals who have been infected with HIV—human immunodeficiency virus. The infection, caused by the virus, weakens the body's immune

Direct Pressure for Bleeding

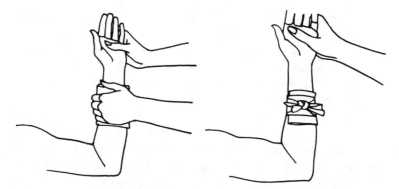

Place a thick sterile or clean compress directly over the entire wound and press firmly with the palm of your hand. If the wound is bleeding severely, elevate the limb above the victim's heart and continue direct pressure.

Once bleeding stops or slows, apply a pressure bandage to hold the compress in place. Place the center of the bandage directly over the compress. Pull steadily while wrapping both ends around the injury. Tie a knot over the compress. *Do not* tie so tightly that it cuts off circulation. Keep the limb elevated.

To apply direct pressure:

1. Place a thick clean compress (sterile gauze or a soft clean cloth such as a handkerchief, towel, undershirt, or strips from a sheet) directly over the entire wound and press firmly with the palm of your hand. (If cloth is not available, use bare hands or fingers, but they should be as clean as possible.)
2. Continue to apply steady pressure.
3. *Do not* disturb any blood clots that form on the compress.
4. If blood soaks through the compress, *do not* remove the compress but apply another pad over it and continue with firmer hand pressure over a wider area.

---

system, rendering the individual "immune-deficient." Over time, the body becomes unable to fight off disease.

AIDS can be passed to others through an infected person's blood and semen. The AIDS virus may be present in saliva, but cases in which AIDS has been transmitted through saliva are unknown at the present time.

You may be aware that those *who regularly come in contact with a patient's or victim's blood or saliva*—doctors, paramedics, other emergency room personnel, and dentists—have begun wearing protective face masks and gloves. *Even among these health-care professionals, the risk of contracting AIDS is very low.*

5. A limb that is bleeding severely should be raised above the level of the victim's heart and direct pressure continued.
6. If bleeding stops or slows, apply a pressure bandage to hold the compress snugly in place.
7. To apply a pressure bandage, place the center of the gauze, cloth strips, or necktie directly over the compress. Pull steadily while wrapping both ends around the injury. Tie a knot over the compress.
9. *Do not* wrap the bandage so tightly that it cuts off arterial circulation. A pulse can be felt on an artery. (Arteries carry blood away from the heart to the extremities.) You should feel a pulse *below* the bandage. (*Note:* "Below" means at a point on an artery that is farthest away from the trunk of the body.)
10. Keep the limb elevated.

II. Pressure Points

Pressure points should be used *only* if bleeding does not stop after the application of direct pressure and elevation. This technique presses the artery supplying blood to the wound against the underlying bone and cuts off arterial circulation to the affected area. Pressure points are used in conjunction with direct pressure and elevation of the wound above the heart.

To apply a pressure point to stop severe bleeding from the *arm*:

1. Grasp the victim's arm bone midway between the armpit and the elbow with your thumb on the outside of the victim's arm and with the flat surface of your fingers on the inside of the arm, where you may actually feel the artery pulsating.
2. Squeeze your fingers firmly toward your thumb against the arm bone until the bleeding stops.

To apply a pressure point to stop severe bleeding from the *leg*:

1. Lay the victim on his or her back, if possible.
2. Place the heel of your hand on the front center part of the thigh, at the crease of the groin. Press down firmly. *Do not* continue the pressure point technique any longer than necessary to stop the bleeding. However, if bleeding recurs, the technique should again be applied.

Pressure Points on the Body and Head

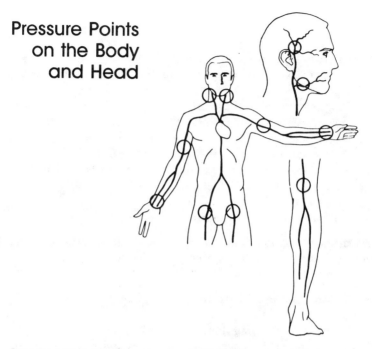

Pressure points should be used *only* if bleeding does not stop after the application of direct pressure and elevation.

III. Tourniquet

WARNING: Use a tourniquet only in life-threatening situations, when severe bleeding cannot be stopped by direct pressure on the wound or by direct pressure on a pressure point. In emergencies, such as partial or complete amputation, where the victim is in danger of bleeding to death, the risk of losing a limb is secondary to saving his or her life.

To apply a tourniquet:

1. The tourniquet should be 2 or more inches wide and long enough to wrap around the limb twice, with ends for tying. A strip of cloth, belt, tie, scarf, or other flat material can be used.
2. Place the tourniquet just above the wound (between the wound and the body) but not touching the wound. Wrap it twice around the limb.
3. Tie a half knot.

4. Place a stick, pen, or other strong, straight object on top of the half knot.
5. Tie two full knots over the stick.
6. Twist the stick to tighten the tourniquet until the bleeding stops.
7. Tie the loose ends of the tourniquet around the stick to hold it in place. Another method of securing the stick is to use a second strip of cloth or other material to tie around the free end of the stick. Then tie the cloth around the limb.
8. *Do not* loosen or remove tourniquet once it has been applied.
9. Attach a note to victim's clothing stating your location and the time the tourniquet was applied.
10. *Do not* cover the tourniquet.

Seek medical attention immediately for any injury that is bleeding severely, particularly when a tourniquet has been applied.

Continued Care Treat for *shock* (p. 237).

1. Keep the victim lying down.
2. Elevate the victim's feet 8 to 12 inches unless the victim is unconscious or has neck, spine, head, chest, severe lower face, or jaw injuries. He or she should be placed on his or her side with the head slightly extended backward (jaws opened) to prevent choking on fluids or vomit. If the victim is having trouble breathing, raise the head and shoulders slightly, keeping the airway clear.
3. If pain increases, lower the feet again unless this makes the victim more uncomfortable.
4. Keep the victim comfortably warm with a blanket or coat, but not too warm. If possible, place a blanket beneath the victim on the ground.
5. If medical attention is more than two hours away, give the victim water or a weak solution of salt (1 level teaspoon) and baking soda (½ level teaspoon) mixed with 1 quart of cool water. Give an adult 4 ounces (½ glass), a child 1 through 12 years 2 ounces, and an infant 1 ounce. Have the victim sip slowly over a 15-minute period. Clear juices, such as apple juice, may also be given.
   Do not give fluids if the victim is unconscious, having convulsions, is likely to need surgery, has a head injury or an abdominal wound, or is vomiting. Stop giving fluids if vomiting occurs.

6. Look for other injuries such as internal bleeding or broken bones and treat them. (See Broken Bones, pp. 93–107.) Treating the injury may lessen the shock.
7. If possible, obtain information about the accident.
8. Calm and reassure the victim. Gentleness, kindness, and understanding play an important role in treating a victim in shock.

INTERNAL BLEEDING

Internal bleeding is not always obvious. You may suspect internal bleeding if the victim has been in an accident, fallen, or received a severe body blow.

Symptoms   Any or all of the following may be present:

1. Vomit that resembles coffee grounds or is red in color.
2. Coughed-up blood that is bright red and/or frothy (bubbly).
3. Stools that are black or contain bright red blood.
4. Paleness.
5. Cold, clammy skin.
6. Rapid and weak pulse.
7. Lightheadedness.
8. Distended (swollen) abdomen.
9. Restlessness.
10. Thirst.
11. Apprehension.
12. Mental confusion.

Immediate   1. Maintain an open airway. Restore breathing, if
Treatment   necessary.
             2. Seek medical attention promptly.

ABCs

With all serious injuries, check and maintain an open airway. Restore breathing (p. 20) and circulation (p. 22), if necessary.

INJURIES AND ILLNESSES

Continued
Care

1. Treat for shock. (See treatment for shock under Continued Care for External Bleeding, p. 84.)
2. *Do not* give the victim anything to drink.
3. Look for other injuries such as broken bones and treat them.
4. Calm and reassure the victim.

NOSEBLEEDS

A nosebleed can be caused by a blow to the nose, scratching the nose, repeated nose blowing that irritates the mucous membrane, or by an infection. Most nosebleeds that occur in children are not serious. Those that occur in the elderly, however, may be serious and may require treatment at a hospital emergency room.

What to Do

1. Have the victim sit down and lean forward, keeping the mouth open so that blood or clots will not obstruct the airway.
2. Squeeze the sides of the nose together for approximately 15 minutes by the clock. (Squeeze the nose below the bone, not on the top of the nose.) Release slowly. *Do not* allow the victim to blow or touch the nose. If bleeding continues, squeeze the nose closed again for 5 minutes. Be sure that the victim is not swallowing blood.
3. Place a cold cloth or ice in a cloth against the victim's nose and face to help constrict blood vessels.
4. If bleeding continues, seek medical attention.
5. Seek medical attention if an injury is involved or if you suspect a broken nose.
6. *Do not* let the victim irritate or blow the nose for several hours after bleeding stops.

See Also: Pregnancy, Danger Signs, p. 221; Severed Limb, p. 232; Shock, p. 237; Wounds, p. 257.

BLISTERS

Blisters are usually caused by clothing (such as shoes) or equipment repeatedly rubbing against the skin.

What to Do

1. If the blister is small and unopened, and will receive no further irritation, cover it with a sterile gauze pad and bandage in place. The fluid in the blister will eventually be absorbed by the skin and it will heal itself.
2. If the blister accidentally breaks, exposing raw skin, wash the area gently with soap and water and cover with a sterile bandage. The skin will regrow its outer layers.
3. *Do not* open a blister that was caused by a burn.
4. If the blister is large and likely to be broken by routine activity, you should seek medical attention for treatment. Only if medical attention is not readily available should you try to open the blister.
5. Gently clean the area with soap and water. Sterilize a needle by holding it over an open flame. Puncture the lower edge of the blister with the needle. Press the blister gently to force out fluid. Cover the area with a sterile bandage.
6. Always look for signs of infection such as redness, pus, or red streaks leading from the wound. Seek medical attention promptly if these symptoms appear.

See Also: Bleeding, p. 80.

BREATHING PROBLEMS IN CHILDREN

Breathing problems in infants and young children are a common occurrence and usually are not serious. However, in some instances, a serious condition does arise that requires immediate medical attention.

CROUP

Croup is a group of symptoms arising from various respiratory conditions in infants and young children. (It is occasionally seen in the older child as well.) Croup is generally caused by a virus, a bacterial infection, or an allergy. Its symptoms occur most often in the fall and end in the spring.

Most attacks of croup occur at night after the child has gone to bed. Often the child has had a mild cold before the attack. Croup that occurs during the day generally becomes more severe in the evening.

Symptoms   Any or all of the following may be present:

1. Difficulty in breathing, particularly inhaling.
2. A croaking sound upon inhaling (called stridor by your doctor).
3. Hoarseness.
4. A hacking, barklike cough.
5. Possible slight fever.
6. Possible bluish tinge to the skin and lips, when the attack is severe.
7. Restlessness.

What to Do   It is important to remain calm during an attack of croup. Reassure the child so that he or she does not become overly frightened. *Do not* place a spoon or other object in the victim's mouth to aid breathing, as this may cause airway obstruction.

To help the child breathe, a cool-mist vaporizer is very helpful and should be placed in the child's room. Or sit with the child in a closed, steam-filled bathroom. (To create steam, let hot water run from the shower or tub for several minutes with the bathroom door closed.) *Do not* put the child in the water. Remain in the bathroom for 20 to 30 minutes. A small child can be held up high where the steam accumulates.

Danger   If symptoms continue and one or more of the fol-
Signals   lowing happens:

1. Worsened condition after the child has been awake a short while.
2. Extreme difficulty in breathing.
3. A croaking sound while inhaling even when the child is calm (called stridor by your doctor).
4. Blue skin and lips.
5. Sudden moderate or high fever.
6. The child becomes agitated or appears exhausted and incapacitated.

WARNING: If the child begins to drool, which may indicate epiglottitis, seek medical attention promptly. Epiglottitis is a *severe* medical condition in which the epiglottis—the flap of tissue at the back of the throat that closes off the windpipe (trachea) during swallowing—becomes inflamed and swells, partially closing off the airway. Call a paramedic unit if one is available or go to the nearest hospital emergency room. *Keep the infant or child in a sitting position.*

EPIGLOTTITIS

Epiglottitis is a serious medical condition in which the epiglottis—the flap of tissue at the back of the throat that closes off the windpipe (trachea) during swallowing—becomes infected, inflamed, and swollen, partially closing off the airway. It usually occurs in children between the ages of 2 and 6. Symptoms may appear after the child has had a severe sore throat or a cold.

Do not place a spoon or other object in the victim's mouth to aid breathing, as this may cause airway obstruction.

A child with any of the symptoms listed below should be treated by paramedics or taken *without delay* to a hospital emergency room.

Symptoms   Any or all of the following may be present:

1. The child has difficulty swallowing.
2. The child drools.
3. The child is quiet, with little or no voice.
4. The child sits straight up with jaw thrust forward in an attempt to keep the airway open.

Immediate Treatment   Call paramedics or take the child *without delay* to a hospital emergency room. *Keep the child in a sitting position.*

UPPER AIRWAY OBSTRUCTION

Occasionally, children will swallow a small object or piece of food—usually popcorn, peanuts, or a bite of a hot dog—that lodges in the upper airway above or between the vocal cords. The lodged object may cause the child's voice to sound strained or strangely mechanical.

What to Do
1. If a piece of food or other object becomes lodged in the child's throat and the child is able to cough or is breathing noisily, he or she will make involuntary attempts to cough out the object.
2. Watch the child carefully and remain as calm as possible so that you do not frighten him or her.
3. *Do not* interfere with the child's efforts to cough out the object.
4. *Do not* stick your fingers down the child's throat, as this may cause the object to become lodged even farther.

5. If the child is unable to cough out the lodged particle, take him or her to a doctor's office or hospital emergency room. Stay with the child at all times, remain calm, and provide reassurance.

Danger Signals   If symptoms continue and one or more of the following happens:

1. The child has extreme difficulty in breathing.
2. The child's skin and lips are blue.
3. The child begins choking.

WARNING: If the infant or child grabs at the throat (an involuntary movement that means he or she is choking) perform the Heimlich maneuver immediately!

Heimlich Maneuver on a Child

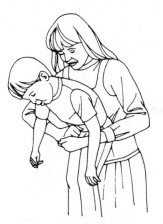

1. If the child cannot breathe, stand behind him or her and place your fist with the thumb side against the child's stomach slightly above the navel and below the ribs and breastbone.

2. Hold your fist with your other hand and give 4 quick, forceful upward thrusts.

3. Do not squeeze on the ribs with your arms. Just use your fist in the abdomen. It may be necessary to repeat the Heimlich maneuver 6 to 10 times.

Heimlich Maneuver on an Infant

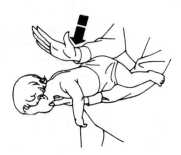

1.) Place the infant or small child face down across your forearm with his or her head low. Support the head by firmly holding the jaw.

2.) Rest your forearm on your thigh and give 4 forceful back blows with the heel of your hand between the shoulder blades.

3.) If unsuccessful, turn the infant over and give 4 quick thrusts on the chest. To do this, place two fingers one finger-width below an imaginary line joining the nipples. Push downward and forward. Thrusts should be more gentle than those for an adult.

4.) If necessary, repeat both procedures.

See Also: Asthma, p. 61.

BROKEN BONES AND SPINAL INJURIES

BROKEN BONES

A break or crack in a bone is a fracture. A fracture may be closed or open. In a **closed fracture,** the broken bone does not come through the skin. Usually the skin is not broken near the fracture site.

In an **open fracture,** there is an open wound that extends down to the bone, or parts of the broken bone may stick out through the skin. An open break is usually more serious because of severe bleeding and the greater possibility of infection.

WARNING: *Do not* move the victim, particularly if he or she has head, neck, or spine injuries (or if paramedics or other trained ambulance personnel are readily available), unless the victim is in immediate danger such as fire, drowning, explosion, gas inhalation, or traffic. If the victim must be moved, immobilize the injured part first. For example, tie the injured leg to the uninjured leg, if possible.

Symptoms   Always suspect a broken bone if any of these symptoms appear:

1. The victim felt or heard a bone snap.
2. The site of the injury is painful or tender, particularly to the touch or when the affected part is moved.
3. There is difficulty in moving the injured part (though the bone may be broken even if the victim can easily move the injured part).
4. The injured part moves abnormally or unnaturally.
5. The victim feels a grating sensation of bone ends rubbing together.

6. The area of the injury is swollen.
7. The injured part is deformed.
8. The shape or length of a bone is different from the same bone on the other side of the body.
9. The site of the injury shows a bluish discoloration.

Immediate Treatment   Follow these procedures with any broken bone or spinal injury:

ABCs

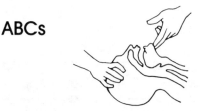

With all serious injuries, check and maintain an open airway. Restore breathing (p. 20) and circulation (p. 22), if necessary.

1. Maintain an open airway. Restore breathing and circulation (pp. 20–22), if necessary. (See Head and Neck Injuries, pp. 188–195, for specific instructions.)
2. Stop any severe bleeding. If the victim has an open break, cut clothing away from the wound.
3. Always suspect a broken neck or spinal injury if the victim is unconscious or has a head injury, neck pain, tingling, or paralysis in the arms or legs. (See Head and Neck Injuries, pp. 188–195.)
4. *Do not* try to push back any part of the bone that is sticking out.
5. *Do not* wash the wound or insert anything, including medication, into it.
6. *Gently* apply pressure with a large sterile or clean pad or cloth to stop the bleeding.
7. Cover the entire wound, including the protruding bone, with a bandage. Splinting an open break is the same as for a closed break. (See Splinting and Other Procedures, p. 95.)
8. Treat for shock (p. 237). See specific types of broken bones on the following pages for information about moving the victim.

9. Call paramedics or an ambulance promptly.

Do not lift a victim with a suspected neck or spinal injury out of the water without a back support, such as a board. If the victim must be dragged to safety, *do not* drag him or her sideways but pull by the armpits or legs in the direction of the length of the body, *keeping the head in line with the body.*

Do not let the victim's body bend or twist, particularly the neck or back. (See Head and Neck Injuries, pp. 188–195.)

10. Apply splints if paramedics or other trained personnel are not readily available and someone else must take the victim to the hospital. Always splint the injured part by securing the splint above and below the injury before moving the victim. (See Splinting and Other Procedures, below.)

11. Handle the victim very gently. Rough handling often increases the severity of the injury.

12. *Do not* give the victim anything to eat or drink.

SPLINTING AND OTHER PROCEDURES

Splints are used to keep an injured part from moving. They ease pain, prevent the break from becoming worse, and help to prevent shock.

Objects that can be used for splinting include boards, straight sticks, brooms, pieces of corrugated cardboard bent to form a three-sided box, rolled newspapers or magazines, pillows, rolled blankets, oars, or umbrellas. The splint should extend beyond both the joint above and the joint below the broken bone.

Padding, such as cloth, towels, or blankets, should be placed between the splint and the skin of the injured part.

Splints can be tied in place with neckties, strips of cloth torn from shirts, handkerchiefs, belts, string, rope, or other suitable material.

Do not tie the splint so tightly that the ties interfere with circulation. Swelling or bluish discoloration in the fingers or toes may indicate that the ties are too tight and need to be loosened. Also loosen splint ties if the victim experiences numbness or tingling or if he or she cannot move the fingers or toes. Check for a pulse and loosen the ties if no pulse can be felt.

Following are instructions on how to splint and treat breaks of specific bones:

INJURIES AND ILLNESSES

Ankle

What to Do
1. Keep the victim lying down.
2. Remove the victim's shoe.
3. Place a pillow (preferably) or rolled blanket around the leg from the calf to well beyond the heel so that the pillow edges meet on top of the leg.
4. Tie the pillow in place.
5. Fold the ends of the pillow that extend beyond the heel so that it supports the foot.

Ankle Injury

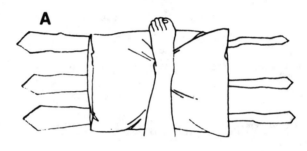

A

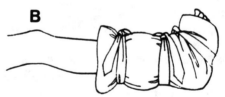

B

A. Remove the victim's shoe. Place a pillow or rolled blanket and ties around the leg from the calf to well beyond the heel.
B. Tie the splint in place. Fold the ends of the pillow that extend beyond the heel so that it supports the foot.

Upper Arm

What to Do
1. Place some light padding in the victim's armpit.
2. Gently place the arm at the victim's side, with the lower part of the arm at a right angle across the victim's chest.
3. Make a padded splint out of newspaper or other material.

Upper Arm Injury

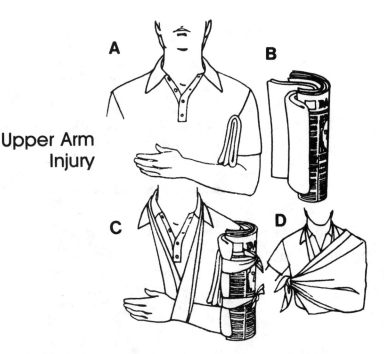

A. Place light padding in the victim's armpit. Then place the arm at the victim's side, with the lower part of the arm at a right angle across the victim's chest.
B. Using newspaper, make a padded splint.
C. Place the padded splint on the outside of the upper arm and tie it in place above and below the break. Support the lower arm with a narrow sling tied around the neck.
D. Bind the upper arm to the victim's body by placing a large towel or other material around the splint and the victim's chest and tying it under the opposite arm.

4. Apply the padded splint to the outside of the upper arm and tie it in place above and below the break.
5. Support the lower arm with a narrow sling tied around the neck.
6. Bind the upper arm to the victim's body by placing a large towel, bedsheet, or cloth around the splint and the victim's chest and tying it under the opposite arm.
7. The victim is usually more comfortable sitting up while riding to the hospital.

Lower Arm and Wrist

What to Do   1.   Carefully place the lower arm at a right angle across the victim's chest with the palm facing toward the chest and the thumb pointing upward.

2.   Apply a padded splint on each side of the lower arm, or use folded, padded newspapers or magazines wrapped under and around both sides of the arm. The splint should reach from the elbow to well beyond the wrist.

Lower Arm or Wrist Injury

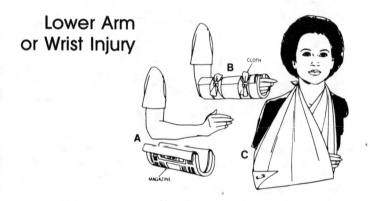

A. Place the lower arm at a right angle across the victim's chest with the palm facing toward the chest and the thumb pointing upward. Apply a padded splint on each side of the lower arm. The splint should reach from the elbow to well beyond the wrist.

B. Tie the splint in place above and below the break.

C. Support the lower arm with a wide sling (see how to apply a sling in Part I, p. 47) tied around the neck. Fingers should be slightly higher (3 to 4 inches) than the level of the elbow.

3.   Tie the splint in place above and below the break.

4.   Support the lower arm with a wide sling tied around the neck. The sling should be placed so that the fingers are slightly higher (3 to 4 inches) than the level of the elbow.

5.   The victim is usually more comfortable sitting up while riding to the hospital.

Back

WARNING: *Never* move a victim with a suspected back injury without trained medical assistance unless the victim is in immediate danger from fire, explosion, or any other life-threatening situation. *Any* movement of the head, neck, or back may result in paralysis or death.

With a severe back or neck injury, the victim may not be able to move the arms, hands, fingers, legs, feet, or toes. The victim may also have tingling, numbness, or pain in the neck or back or down the arms or legs.

What to Do

1. If the victim must be removed from an automobile or from water, immobilize the back and neck with a reasonably short, wide board. The board should reach down to the victim's buttocks.
2. Place the board behind the victim's head, neck, and back, *keeping these body parts in alignment.*
3. Tie the board around the victim's forehead, under the armpits, and around the lower abdomen.
4. *Do not* let the victim's body bend or twist. Move the victim very gently and slowly.
5. If the victim is not breathing, tilt his or her head back *slightly* to maintain an open airway. If the victim is face down, get adequate help so that every part of the body can be turned over together in the same position in which it was found. Restore breathing, if necessary.

(*continued on p. 101*)

INJURIES AND ILLNESSES

ABCs

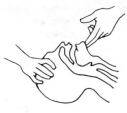

With all serious injuries, check and maintain an open airway. Restore breathing (p. 20) and circulation (p. 22), if necessary.

Mouth-to-Mouth Resuscitation

If the victim is not breathing and no neck injury is suspected, perform all of the following 4 steps.

If a neck injury is suspected (as in a diving or motorcycle accident, or from a fall from a height) *do not* twist or rotate the head. *Slightly* elevate the chin only to open the airway. Check for foreign material in the mouth. Then continue with steps 3 and 4, below.*

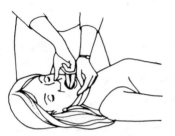

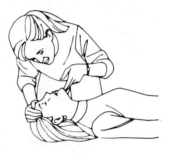

1. Make sure the victim is on a hard, flat surface. Quickly clear the mouth and airway of foreign material.

2. Tilt the victim's head backward by placing the palm of your hand on his or her forehead and the fingers of your other hand under the bony part of the chin.

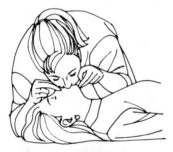

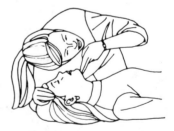

3. Pinch the victim's nostrils with your thumb and index finger. Take a deep breath. Place your mouth tightly over the victim's mouth (mouth and nose for an infant or small child). Give two quick breaths.

4. Stop blowing when the chest is expanding. Remove your mouth from the victim's mouth and turn your head toward the victim's chest, so that your ear is over his or her mouth. *Listen* for air being exhaled. *Watch* for the victim's chest to fall. Repeat breathing procedure.

*To move a victim with a neck injury, see p. 191.

(*continued from p. 99*)

6. Place folded blankets, towels, or clothing at the victim's sides, head, and neck to keep him or her from rotating or moving from side to side.
7. Keep the victim comfortably warm.

*If a victim with a back injury must be taken to the hospital by someone **other** than trained medical personnel:*

What to Do
1. If you are unsure whether the injury is to the neck or the back, treat it as if it were a neck injury. (See Head and Neck Injuries, pp. 188–195.)

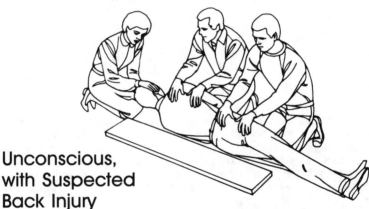

INJURIES AND ILLNESSES

Unconscious, with Suspected Back Injury

If the victim is vomiting or unconscious, transport him or her on the side. Roll the victim over as a unit, keeping the victim's head in the same relationship to the body as it was found. *Do not* let the head move alone. Move the entire body together.

2. A victim with a suspected back injury *must* be taken to the hospital lying down. If the victim is conscious, transport in the position in which the victim was found; that is, face up or face down.

   Do not, however, transport face down if the victim has severe chest or face injuries. If the victim is unconscious, transport him or her on the side to prevent choking on vomit. Roll the victim over as a unit, keeping the head in the same relationship to the body as it was found.

3. Place a well-padded rigid support such as a door, table leaf, or wide board next to the victim.

4. Slide ties under the support.

Suspected Back Injury

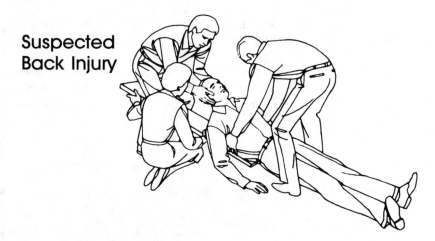

If a victim with a suspected back injury must be taken to the hospital by someone other than trained medical personnel, the victim must be transported lying down. Place well-padded rigid support such as a door next to the victim. The victim's head must be held so that it stays in the same relationship to the body as it was found. Helpers should grasp the victim's clothes and *slide* the victim onto the support. Move the entire body as a unit.

5. If the victim is breathing on his or her own, hold the head so that it does not move but stays in the same relationship to the body as it was found. Other helpers should grasp the victim's clothing and *slide* the victim onto the support. Move the entire body together.

6. Place folded towels, blankets, or clothing at the victim's sides, head, and neck to keep him or her from moving. If the victim is lying on his or her back, place padding in the hollow of the back.

7. Tie or tape the victim's body to the support.

8. Drive carefully to prevent further injury.

Collarbone

What to Do   With an elastic bandage or other cloth, apply a figure-of-eight bandage around the victim's shoulder, back, and chest.

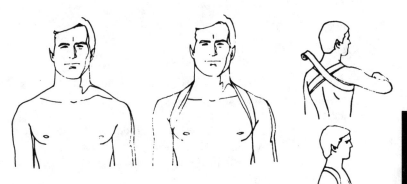

Collarbone Injury

Wrap a bandage (starting under either arm) diagonally across the back, over the shoulder, under the arm and again diagonally across the back, over the shoulder, and under the arm. Repeat a few times. You should be able to slide one finger snugly under the ties in front. Illustration shows front, side, and back views.

Elbow

Elbow fractures often cause circulatory problems. The victim should seek medical help at once if an elbow injury is suspected.

If the elbow is *bent*:

What to Do   1. *Do not* try to straighten the elbow.
2. Place the forearm in a sling and tie the sling around the victim's neck if possible.
3. If possible, bind the injured upper arm to the victim's body by placing a towel or cloth around the upper arm, sling, and chest and tying it under the victim's opposite arm.

If the elbow is *straight*:

What to Do   1. *Do not* try to bend the elbow to apply a sling.
2. Place padding in the victim's armpit.

INJURIES AND ILLNESSES

3. Apply padded splints along one or both sides of the entire arm. If splints are not available, a pillow centered at the elbow and tied may be used.

Foot

See Ankle, p. 96.

Hand

What to Do
1. Place a padded splint underneath the lower arm and hand.
2. Tie the splint in place.
3. Place the lower arm and elbow at a right angle to the victim's chest.
4. Put the lower arm into a sling and tie around the victim's neck.

Hand Injury

A. Place a padded splint underneath the lower arm and hand.
B. Tie the splint in place.
C. Place the lower arm and elbow at a right angle to the victim's chest. Put the lower arm into a sling and tie it around the victim's neck. (See how to apply a sling in Part I, p. 47.)

Kneecap

See Also: Dislocations, p. 147.

What to Do
1. Gently straighten the victim's injured leg, if necessary.

2. Place a padded board at least 4 inches wide underneath the injured leg. The board should be long enough to reach from the victim's heel to the buttocks.
3. Place extra padding under the ankle and knee.
4. Tie the splint in place at the ankle, just below and above the knee, and at the thigh.
   Do not tie over the kneecap.

Kneecap Injury

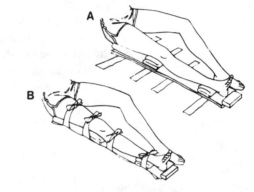

A. Place a padded board at least 4 inches wide underneath the injured leg. The board should reach from the victim's heel to the buttocks. Place extra padding under the ankle and knee.
B. Tie the splint in place at the ankle, just below and above the knee, and at the thigh. *Do not* tie over the kneecap.

Upper Leg (Thigh)

If board splints are *not* available:

What to Do
1. Using traction (pull), carefully and slowly straighten the knee of the injured leg, if necessary.
2. Place padding, such as a folded blanket, between the victim's legs.
3. Tie the injured leg to the uninjured leg. Legs should be tied together in several places, including around the ankles, above and below the knees, and around the thighs.
   Do not tie directly over the break.

If board splints are available:

What to Do
1. Using traction (pull), carefully and slowly straighten the knee of the injured leg if necessary.
2. Assemble about seven long bandages or cloth strips. Use a stick or small board to push each strip under the victim's body at a hollow such as the ankle, knee, or small of the back and then slide each strip into place (at the ankle, above and below the knee, at the thigh, pelvis, and lower back, and just below the armpit).
3. Place two well-padded splints in parallel position. The outside splint should be long enough to reach from the victim's armpit to below the heel. The inside splint should reach from the crotch to below the heel.
4. Tie the splints in place with knots at the outside splint.

Lower Leg

If splints are *not* available:

What to Do
1. Carefully and slowly straighten the injured leg, if necessary.
2. Place padding, such as a folded blanket, between the victim's legs.
3. Tie the legs together. (See Upper Leg, p. 105.)

If splints are available:

What to Do
1. Place a well-padded splint on each side of the injured leg. A third splint can be used underneath the leg. Splints should reach from above the knee to below the heel.
2. Tie the splints together in three or four places. *Do not* tie directly over the break.

To make a pillow splint:

What to Do
1. Gently lift the injured leg and slide the pillow under the leg.
2. Bring the edges of the pillow to the top side of the leg. Pin the pillow together or tie the pillow

around the leg in several places. For added support, place a rigid object such as a board or stick on each side of the pillow and fasten in place with ties above and below the suspected fracture site.

Neck

(See Head and Neck Injuries, pp. 188–195.)

Pelvis

What to Do
1. Keep the victim lying down on his or her back.
2. Legs may be straight or bent at the knees, whichever is more comfortable for the victim.
3. Tie the victim's legs together at the ankles and knees whether the legs are straight or bent.
4. If the victim must be taken to the hospital by someone other than trained medical personnel, place the victim on a well-padded rigid support such as a board, door, or table leaf. (See transporting with a back injury, p. 101.)

Shoulder

What to Do
1. Place the victim's injured forearm at a right angle to his or her chest.
2. Apply a sling and tie around the victim's neck.
3. Bind the arm to the victim's body by placing a towel or cloth around the upper arm and chest and tying it under the victim's opposite arm.
4. The victim is usually more comfortable sitting up while riding to the hospital.

Skull

(See Head and Neck Injuries, pp. 188–195.)

See Also: Bleeding, p. 80; Dislocations, p. 147; Head and Neck Injuries, p. 188; Shock, p. 234; Sprains, p. 243; Wounds, p. 257.

INJURIES AND ILLNESSES

BRUISES

A bruise is the most common type of injury. It occurs when a fall or blow to the body causes small blood vessels to break beneath the skin. The discoloration and swelling in the skin are caused by the blood seeping into the tissues, which change colors as the bruise heals.

Symptoms
1. Pain.
2. Initial reddening of the skin.
3. Later, the bruise turns blue or green in color.
4. Occasionally, a lump called a hematoma forms at the site.
5. Finally, the area becomes brown and yellow before fading.

What to Do
1. As soon as possible apply cold compresses or an ice bag to the affected area. Cold or ice decreases local bleeding and swelling.
2. If bruise is on the arm or leg, elevate the limb above the level of the heart to decrease local blood flow.
3. After 24 hours, apply moist heat (a warm wet compress) to aid healing. Heat dilates or opens blood vessels, increasing circulation to the affected area.
4. If the bruise is severe or painful swelling develops, seek medical attention, as there is the possibility of a broken bone or other injury.

See Also: Bleeding, p. 80; Broken Bones and Spinal Injuries, p. 93; Dislocations, p. 147; Lumps and Bumps, p. 203; Muscle Aches and Pains, p. 208; Sprains, p. 243.

BURNS

The objectives of first aid for burns are to relieve pain, prevent infection, and prevent or treat for shock.

Initial treatment of burns by the first-aider helps to decrease the *temperature* of the burned area. This, in turn, helps prevent further heat injury to the skin and underlying tissues.

Burns caused by *fire, sunlight,* or *hot substances* are classified according to the degree of the injury. First-degree burns are the least dangerous. Third-degree burns are the most serious.

As in all serious injuries, first check and maintain an open airway. Restore breathing and circulation if necessary.

ABCs

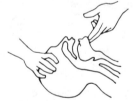

With all serious injuries, check and maintain an open airway. Restore breathing (p. 20) and circulation (p. 22), if necessary.

FIRST-DEGREE BURNS

A burn resulting in injury only to the outside layer of the skin is a first-degree burn. Sunburn and brief contact with hot objects, hot water, or steam are common causes of first-degree burns and cause no blistering of the burned areas.

Symptoms   Any or all of the following may be present:

1. Redness.
2. Mild swelling.
3. Pain.
4. Unbroken skin (no blisters).

What to Do   1.   Immediately put the burned area under cold running water or apply a cold-water compress (a clean towel, washcloth, or handkerchief soaked in cold water) until pain decreases.

2.   Cover burn with nonfluffy sterile or clean bandages.

   Do not apply butter or grease to a burn. Do not apply other medications or home remedies without a doctor's recommendation.

To Treat a Burn

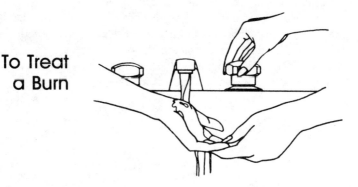

Immediately put the burned area under cold running water (as illustrated) or apply cold-water compresses until pain subsides.

SECOND-DEGREE BURNS

A burn that causes injury to the layers of skin beneath the surface of the body is a second-degree burn. Deep sunburn, hot liquids, and flash burns from gasoline and other substances are common causes of second-degree burns.

Symptoms   Any or all of the following may be present:

1. Redness, or blotchy or streaky appearance of burn.
2. Blisters.

3. Swelling that lasts for several days.
4. Moist, oozy appearance of the surface of the skin.
5. Pain.

What to Do
1. Put the burned area in cold water (not iced) or apply cold-water compresses (a clean towel, washcloth, or handkerchief soaked in cold water) until pain subsides.
2. Gently pat the area dry with a clean towel or other soft material.
3. Cover the burned area with a dry, nonfluffy sterile bandage or clean cloth to prevent infection.
4. Elevate burned arms or legs.
5. Seek medical attention. If the victim has flash burns around the lips or nose, or has singed nasal hairs, breathing problems may develop. Seek medical attention immediately, preferably at the nearest hospital emergency room.
   Do not attempt to break blisters.
   Do not apply ointments, sprays, antiseptics, or home remedies.

NOTE: *Any cold liquid you can drink—such as water, iced tea, a soft drink, beer, or a milk shake—can be poured on a burn. The purpose in doing so is to decrease the temperature of the burned skin* as quickly as possible *so as to limit tissue damage.*

WARNING: Prompt medical attention is required for burns that cover more than 15 percent of the body of an adult or 10 percent of the body of a child, or for burns of the face, hands, or feet. To determine the percentage of the burned area, an easy rule is that your hand (including fingers) represents 1 percent of your body area. Victims who have inhaled smoke or other substances can develop lung damage.

THIRD-DEGREE BURNS

A burn that destroys all layers of the skin is a third-degree burn. Fire, prolonged contact with hot substances, and electrical burns are common causes of third-degree burns.

INJURIES AND ILLNESSES

Symptoms   Any or all of the following may be present:

1. The burned area appears white or charred.
2. Destroyed skin.
3. Little pain is present because nerve endings have been destroyed.

WARNING:

1. *Do not* remove clothes that are stuck to the burn.
2. *Do not* put ice or ice water on burns. This can intensify the shock reaction.
3. *Do not* apply ointments, sprays, antiseptics, or home remedies to burns.

Immediate
Treatment

1. If the victim is on fire, smother the flames with a blanket, bedspread, rug, or jacket.
2. Breathing difficulties are common with burns, particularly with burns around the face, neck, and mouth, and with smoke inhalation. Check to be sure that the victim is breathing.
3. Place a cold cloth or cool (not iced) water on burns of the face, hands, or feet to cool the burned areas.
4. Cover the burned area with thick, sterile, non-fluffy dressings. A clean sheet, pillowcase, or disposable diaper can be used.
5. Call for an ambulance immediately. It is very important that victims with even *small* third-degree burns consult a doctor.

Continued
Care

1. Elevate burned hands higher than the victim's heart, if possible.
2. Elevate burned legs or feet. Do not allow the victim to walk.
3. If the victim has face or neck burns, he or she should be propped up with pillows. Check often to see if the victim has trouble breathing and maintain an open airway if breathing becomes difficult.
4. Treat for shock.
   (a) Keep the victim lying down unless the face or neck is burned.

(b) Elevate the victim's feet 8 to 12 inches unless the victim is unconscious or has neck, spine, head, chest, or severe lower face or jaw injuries. A victim who is unconscious or who has severe lower face or jaw injuries should be placed on his or her side (not face down) with the head slightly extended to prevent choking on fluids or vomit. If the victim is having trouble breathing, elevate his or her head and shoulders slightly.

Elevate a Burn

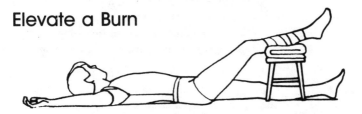

Elevate a foot or leg with second-or third-degree burns higher than the victim's heart.

Cover the burn with a non-fluffy sterile or clean bandage to prevent infection. Elevate a hand or arm with second- or third-degree burns higher than the victim's heart.

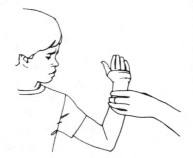

(c) If pain increases, lower the feet again.

(d) Keep the victim comfortably warm but not hot, covered with a blanket or coat. If possible, place a blanket beneath a victim who is on the ground.

(e) If medical attention is more than two hours away, give the victim water or a weak solution of salt (1 level teaspoon) and baking soda (½ level teaspoon), mixed with 1 quart cool water. Give an adult 4 ounces (½ glass), a child 1 through 12 years old 2 ounces, and an infant 1 ounce. Have the victim sip slowly over a 15-minute period and repeat every 15 minutes. Clear juices, such as apple juice, may also be given.

Do not give fluids if the victim is unconscious, having convulsions, is likely to need surgery, has a head injury or an abdominal wound, or is vomiting. Stop giving fluids if vomiting occurs.

(f) *Do not* give the victim alcohol.

(g) Calm and reassure the victim. Gentleness, kindness, and understanding play an important role in treating a victim in shock.

CHEMICAL BURNS

Immediate Treatment

1. Quickly flush the burned area with large quantities of running water for at least five minutes. Speed and quantity of water are both important in minimizing the extent of the injury. Use a garden hose, buckets of water, a shower, or a tub. Do not use a strong stream of water if it can be avoided.

2. Continue to flush with water while removing clothing from the burned area.

3. After flushing, follow instructions on label of the chemical that caused the burn, if available.

4. Cover the burn with a nonfluffy clean bandage or clean cloth.

5. Seek medical attention, but treat first as directed above. *Do not* apply ointments, sprays, antiseptics, or home remedies. Cool wet dressings are best for pain.

See Also: Convulsions, p. 133; Electric Shock, p. 166; Overexposure: Heat and Cold, p. 209; Shock, p. 234.

CHILD ABUSE (MISUSE)/OTHER PERSON ABUSE

Reported cases of child abuse, and abuse of other individuals, such as spouses and the elderly, have risen dramatically. Abuse can take many forms—emotional, mental, physical, or sexual.

In most instances the abuser is a parent or other family member, a relative, a neighbor, or some other adult. People who abuse oftentimes have been abused themselves.

Making an assessment that child abuse or other personal abuse has occurred or is occurring can be difficult. Always call the police if you suspect *with good reason* that a child or other person is being abused or is in danger of losing his or her life. If you are abusing a child or other person, help is available for you. Call a child abuse hotline or other community agency that offers counseling.

Symptoms   Some symptoms and signs of abuse are more obvious than others. If a child has been physically abused, he or she may exhibit or have the following:

1. Frequent complaints of pain.
2. Frequently broken bones.
3. Cuts, bruises, or burn marks.
4. Bleeding.
5. An unkempt appearance.
6. Is withdrawn, depressed, or inattentive.
7. Is *overly* aggressive, especially with other children or siblings.

If sexual abuse is suspected, the child may have the following symptoms and signs:

1. Complaints of pain when urinating.
2. *Unusual* fear of adults.

3. Is *overly* pleasing to adults and others.
4. An unkempt appearance.
5. Is withdrawn, depressed, or inattentive.
6. Is *overly* aggressive, especially with other children or siblings.
7. Shows other signs of abuse (cuts, bruises, or burn marks).

Immediate Treatment If you are in a situation in which you can help a victim of abuse, offer assistance in treating noticeable injuries, such as cuts, bruises, or burns.

1. If the victim is unconscious, restore breathing and circulation, if necessary.

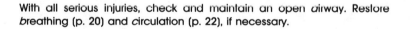

With all serious injuries, check and maintain an open airway. Restore *breathing* (p. 20) and *circulation* (p. 22), if necessary.

2. Stop any severe bleeding. (See Bleeding, p. 80.)
3. Treat any broken bones. (See Broken Bones, p. 93.)
4. Treat for symptoms of shock. (See Shock, p. 234.)
5. Comfort the victim as much as possible.

If a child or other person has suffered any of these serious injuries, take him or her to a doctor's office or hospital emergency room *without delay* for further treatment. Do not wash the child or allow the child to take a shower or bath.

(*continued on p. 118*)

Mouth-to-Mouth Resuscitation

If the victim is not breathing and no neck injury is suspected, perform the following 4 steps.

If a neck injury is suspected (as in a diving or motorcycle accident, or from a fall from a height) *do not* twist or rotate the head. *Slightly* elevate the chin only to open the airway. Check for foreign material in the mouth. Then continue with steps 3 and 4, below.*

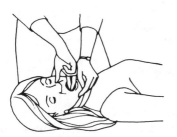

1.) Make sure the victim is on a hard, flat surface. Quickly clear the mouth and airway of foreign material.

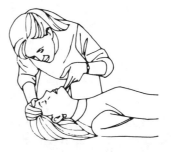

2.) Tilt the victim's head backward by placing the palm of your hand on his or her forehead and the fingers of your other hand under the bony part of the chin.

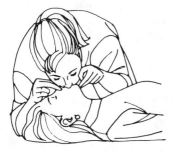

3.) Pinch the victim's nostrils with your thumb and index finger. Take a deep breath. Place your mouth tightly over the victim's mouth (mouth and nose for an infant or small child).

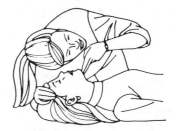

4.) Stop blowing when the chest is expanding. Remove your mouth from the victim's mouth and turn your head toward the victim's chest, so that your ear is over his or her mouth. *Listen* for air being exhaled. *Watch* for the victim's chest to fall. Repeat the breathing procedure.

*To move a victim with a neck injury, see page 191.

(continued from p. 116)

Do Not Allow the Victim to:

| Change clothes. | Take a shower. | Brush his or her teeth. |

Do the Following:

Call the police to report the crime.

Call someone to assist you: a relative or friend.

Call your doctor or hospital emergency room.

When you seek medical treatment for the victim, he or she will be given a private room or a secluded area at the physician's office or hospital emergency room. A counselor, policeman or policewoman, and medical personnel may all be present to help the child or other person. You or the victim may be asked to describe several times what happened and to give a description of the assailant.

A physician will recommend that the victim have a complete physical examination. The exam is performed to protect the child or other person from disease and to support possible criminal charges of rape or other physical abuse.

The exam will include taking cultures (samples) from the mouth, vagina, and rectum, tests for infections (i.e., chlamydia, gonorrhea, syphilis), for pregnancy, and, possibly, for AIDS. The tests will determine the victim's health status for these conditions at the time the crime occurred.

Continued Care

1. Have someone stay with the victim. Do not allow the victim to stay alone.
2. If you are taking care of a rape victim, offer your support.
3. The victim will be requested to seek follow-up medical treatment, depending upon the injuries and test results.
4. Medical personnel may advise the victim to seek counseling for assistance in handling the emotional aspects of physical abuse or of rape.

CHILDBIRTH, EMERGENCY

Occasionally childbirth occurs at an unexpected time or labor proceeds more quickly than expected. In such cases, the mother sometimes cannot get to the hospital in time for the delivery of the infant.

If the mother's contractions are two to three minutes apart, if she feels the urge to push down or to move her bowels, or if the baby's head is visible (about the size of a half-dollar or larger) in the vaginal opening, birth will usually occur very soon.

If at all possible, summon a doctor to deliver the infant. Sometimes a doctor can give instructions over the telephone during the delivery.

Try to remain calm. Most births occur naturally and normally.

Do not try to delay or prevent the birth of the baby by crossing the mother's legs or pushing on the baby's head or by any other means. This could be very harmful to the infant.

PREPARATION AND DELIVERY

Before the Baby Arrives

What to Do
1. Place clean sheets on the bed. If time allows, a shower curtain or rubber sheet placed underneath the clean linen will help protect the mattress. If no bed is readily available, place clean cloths, clothes, or newspapers underneath the mother's hips and thighs on the floor or ground. A fresh newspaper is generally very clean and almost sterile.
2. Have the mother lie on her back with her knees bent, her feet flat, and her knees and

thighs wide apart. If the mother is on a bed, leave enough room for the birth of the baby.

3. Wash your hands with soap and water.

Preparation for Birth

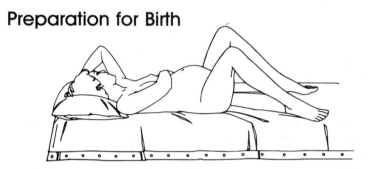

Place clean sheets on the bed. If no bed is available, place clean cloths, clothes, or newspapers underneath the mother's hips and thighs on the floor. Leaving room for the birth of the baby, have the mother lie on her back with her knees bent, her feet flat, and her knees and thighs wide apart.

4. Sterilize scissors or a knife in boiling water for at least 5 minutes if possible or hold over a flame for 30 seconds. Leave the scissors in the water until you are ready to use them. The scissors may be used to cut the umbilical cord.

5. Gather together:
    (a) A clean, soft cotton blanket, sheet, or towel to wrap the baby in after it is born.
    (b) Clean, strong string, clean shoelaces, cord, or strips of cloth to be used to tie off the umbilical cord.
    (c) A pail or bucket to be used if the mother vomits.
    (d) A large plastic bag, container, or towel in which to place the afterbirth (placenta) for later inspection by medical personnel.
    (e) Sanitary napkins or clean folded cloths or handkerchiefs to be placed over the vagina after the birth of the baby and the delivery of the afterbirth.
    (f) Diapers and safety pins.

Delivering the Baby

What to Do
1. *Do not* place your hands or other objects in the vagina.
2. *Do not* interfere with the delivery or touch the baby until the head is completely out of the vagina.
3. Once the baby's head is out, guide and support it to keep it free of blood and other secretions.
4. If the baby's head is still inside a liquid-filled bag, *carefully* puncture the bag with the sterile scissors or your finger and open it to allow the fluid to escape. Remove the membranes from the baby's face so that the baby can breathe.
5. Usually the baby will be born facedown. Check to make sure the umbilical cord is not wrapped around the baby's neck. If it is, gently and quickly slip the cord over the baby's head.
6. If the cord is wrapped too tightly to slip over the baby's head, the cord must be cut *now* to prevent the baby from choking. This is a *rare occurrence,* however.

    If you have cut the cord and if someone is available to help you, have that individual tie off the umbilical cord ends. (See Immediate Care of the Baby, number 8, p. 123.)

    If the umbilical cord is *not* wrapped around the baby's neck, do not worry about cutting the cord until after the baby's birth.
7. Continue to support the head as the baby is being born. The baby will be very slippery, so be gentle and very careful.
8. Once the baby's head and neck are out of the vagina, the baby will turn himself or herself on his or her side (facing the mother's thighs) to allow for the birth of the shoulders. The upper shoulder usually passes first. *Carefully* and *gently* guide the baby's head slightly downward. Once the upper shoulder is out, *gently* lift the baby's head upward to allow the lower shoulder to emerge.

INJURIES AND ILLNESSES

9. Carefully hold the slippery baby as the rest of his or her body slides out.

Immediate Care of the Baby

What to Do

To help the baby start breathing, hold the baby with his or her head lower than the feet so that secretions can drain from the lungs, mouth, and nose. Support the head and body with one hand while grasping the baby's legs at the ankles with the other hand.

2. Wipe out the mouth and nose gently with sterile gauze or a clean cloth to make sure that nothing interferes with breathing.
3. If the baby has not yet cried, slap your fingers against the bottom of the baby's feet or gently rub the baby's back.
4. If the baby is still not breathing, give artificial respiration through *both* the baby's mouth and nose, keeping the head extended. (See p. 20.) Give very gentle puffs every 3 seconds.
5. Note the time of delivery.

After the Birth

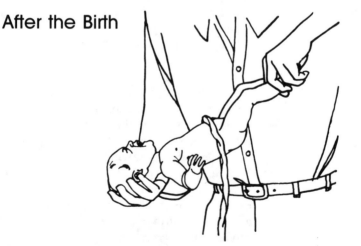

After the baby is born, hold the baby with his or her head lower than the feet so that secretions can drain from the lungs, mouth, and nose. Support the head and body with one hand while grasping the baby's legs and ankles with the other hand.

6. Once the baby starts breathing, to prevent heat loss, wrap the infant, including the top and back of his or her head, in a blanket or sheet. Place the baby on his or her side on the mother's stomach with the baby's head slightly lower than the rest of the body. The baby should be facing the mother's feet. The umbilical cord should be kept slack. It is very important that the baby be kept warm and breathing well.

   Do not clean the white cheesy coating covering the baby's skin. This is a protective covering. *Do not* clean the baby's eyes or ears.

7. It is not necessary or desirable to cut the umbilical cord immediately. It is best to wait about five minutes, until the cord stops pulsating. If the mother can be taken to the hospital immediately after the delivery of the afterbirth (placenta), the baby can be left attached to the umbilical cord and afterbirth, particularly if there are no clean scissors to cut the cord. Also, the cord must be cut properly.

8. If you must cut the cord, tie a clean string or strip of cloth around the cord at least 4 inches from the baby's body. Tie the string in a tight square knot so that circulation is cut off in the

Tying the Umbilical Cord

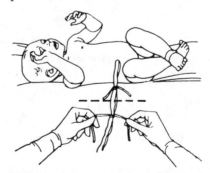

If the umbilical cord is to be cut, tie a clean string around the cord at least 4 inches from the baby's body. Tie in a *tight* square knot so that circulation is cut off in the cord. Use a second piece of string to tie another *tight* square knot 6 to 8 inches from the baby (2 to 4 inches from the first knot) toward the mother. Cut the cord *between* the two ties.

cord. Using a second piece of string or strip of cloth, tie another *tight* square knot 6 to 8 inches from the baby (2 to 4 inches from the first knot) toward the mother.

9. Cut the cord *between* the two ties with sterilized or clean scissors or knife.

10. Keep the baby warm with his or her head covered and close to the mother. The baby's head should still be slightly lower than the rest of his or her body to allow for drainage of secretions.

DELIVERY OF THE AFTERBIRTH

Delivery of the afterbirth (placenta) usually occurs within 5 to 20 minutes after the birth of the baby. It is usually preceded by a gush of dark red blood from the vagina.

What to Do
1. Be patient in waiting for the delivery of the afterbirth.

2. *Do not* pull on the umbilical cord to quicken delivery of the afterbirth. The mother's uterine contractions will eventually push out the afterbirth.

3. There will be bleeding with the delivery of the baby and the afterbirth.

4. Place the afterbirth in a container and take it with the mother and the baby to the hospital (preferably) or other medical facility so that it may be examined.

CARE OF THE MOTHER

After the infant has been born and the afterbirth is expelled:

1. Place sanitary napkins or other clean folded cloths against the mother's vaginal opening to absorb blood.

2. To help control the flow of blood from the mother, place your hands on the mother's abdomen and gently massage the uterus, which can be felt just below the mother's navel and feels like a

large smooth ball. Continue to massage gently until the uterus feels *firm*. Continue to do this every 5 minutes or so for an hour, unless medical assistance is obtained sooner. If the bleeding is very heavy and/or prolonged, seek medical attention immediately.
3. Sponge the mother's face with cool water if she wishes.
4. Give the mother water, tea, coffee, or broth, if she desires something to drink. *Do not* give her alcoholic beverages.
5. Keep the mother warm and comfortable. And remember, congratulations are in order!

MEDICAL ATTENTION

Regardless of how smoothly the delivery goes, it is very important that both the mother and the baby be examined by a physician to make certain all is well. Most serious problems occur in the first 24 hours after birth.

See Also: Miscarriage, p. 207; Pregnancy, Danger Signs, p. 221.

INJURIES AND ILLNESSES

CHILLS

Chills may be a symptom of flu, kidney and bladder infections, bacterial pneumonia, salmonella food poisoning, brown recluse spider bites, or many other medical problems.

Chills are also associated with exposure to cold. (See Overexposure: Heat and Cold, p. 209.)

Chills are nature's way of raising the body temperature. Chills occur when there is decreased blood circulation to the body surface due to narrowing of the blood vessels in the skin. Muscles in the body also contract. Shivering and shaking associated with chills produce heat in the body, thus allowing the body temperature to rise. Often, chills are followed by fever and indicate the onset of an infectious process.

Make the victim comfortably warm. Do not use hot water bottles or heating pads. Warm drinks and liquids such as tea or soup are also helpful if the victim is not nauseated or vomiting. It is advisable to seek medical attention, as a serious infection may be present.

See Also: Bites and Stings (Spider Bites), p. 68; Fever, p. 177; Food Poisoning, p. 183; Overexposure: Heat and Cold, p. 209.

CHOKING

Heimlich Maneuver (Abdominal Thrust)

The Heimlich maneuver (abdominal thrust) is the method of choice to use in an emergency situation when a person is choking. Back blows—hitting the victim forcefully and repeatedly between the shoulder blades with the palm of your hand—are used on adults and children only if the Heimlich maneuver has not been effective in dislodging a foreign object from the windpipe (trachea).

Symptoms

1. The victim begins gasping or breathing noisily.
2. The victim grasps his or her throat.
3. The victim is unable to talk.
4. The victim has difficulty in breathing and begins coughing; breathing may stop.
5. The skin becomes pale, white, gray, or blue.
6. The victim looks or acts panicked.
7. Unconsciousness eventually develops.

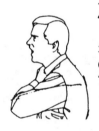

The Universal Choking Sign

A person who is choking will involuntarily grasp his or her neck.

For an Adult or a Child:

Immediate Treatment

If the Victim Is Conscious:

1. If the victim can speak, cough, or breathe (meaning that he or she is moving air through the airway), do not interfere in any way with his or her efforts to cough out a swallowed or partially swallowed object.

2.   If the victim cannot breathe, stand behind him or her and place your fist with the thumb side against the victim's stomach slightly above the navel and below the ribs and breastbone. Hold your fist with your other hand and give 4 quick, forceful upward thrusts. This maneuver increases pressure in the abdomen, which pushes up the diaphragm. This, in turn, increases the air pressure in the lungs and will often force out the object from the windpipe.

Do not squeeze on the ribs with your arms. Just use your fist in the abdomen. It may be necessary to repeat the Heimlich maneuver 6 to 10 times.

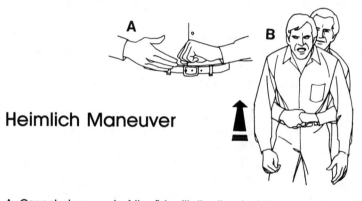

Heimlich Maneuver

A. Correct placement of the fist, with the thumb side against the victim's stomach slightly above the navel and below the ribs and breastbone.
B. If the victim is standing or sitting, stand behind the victim with your arms around his or her waist. Place your fist as shown in the illustration. Hold your fist with your other hand and give 4 quick, forceful upward thrusts.

3.   If the victim is lying down, turn the victim on his or her back. Straddle the victim and put the heel of your hand on the victim's stomach, slightly above the navel and below the ribs. Put your free hand on top of your other hand to provide additional force. Keep your elbows straight. Give 4 quick, forceful downward and forward thrusts toward the head in an attempt to dislodge the object. Doing so will increase pressure in the abdomen, forcing pressure into the lungs to expel the object out of the windpipe and into the mouth.

It may be necessary to repeat the procedure 6 to 10 times.

4.   If you get no results, repeat the Heimlich maneuver until the victim coughs up the object or becomes unconscious. Look to

(continued on p. 130)

Mouth-to-Mouth Resuscitation

If the victim is not breathing and no neck injury is suspected, perform all of the following 4 steps.

If a neck injury is suspected (as in a diving or motorcycle accident,
or from a fall from a height) *do not* twist or rotate the head. *Slightly*
elevate the chin only to open the airway. Check for foreign material
in the mouth. Then continue with steps 3 and 4, below.*

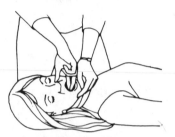

1. Make sure the victim is on a
hard, flat surface. Quickly clear
the mouth and airway of foreign material.

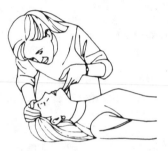

2. Tilt the victim's head backward
by placing the palm of your
hand on his or her forehead
and the fingers of your other
hand under the bony part of
the chin.

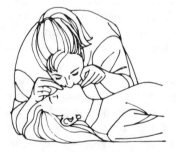

3. Pinch the victim's nostrils with
your thumb and index finger.
Take a deep breath. Place
your mouth tightly over the victim's mouth (mouth and nose
for an infant or small child).
Give 2 quick breaths.

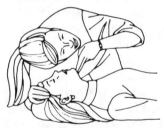

4. Stop blowing when the chest
is expanding. Remove your
mouth from the victim's mouth
and turn your head toward the
victim's chest, so that your ear
is over his or her mouth. *Listen*
for air being exhaled. *Watch*
for the victim's chest to fall. Repeat the breathing procedure.

*To move a victim with a neck injury, see p. 191.

INJURIES AND ILLNESSES

Heimlich Maneuver on a Victim Lying Down

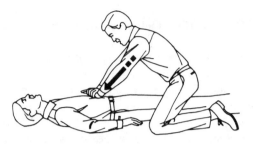

Straddle the victim and put the heel of your hand on the victim's stomach, slightly above the navel and below the ribs. Put your free hand on top of your other hand. Keep your elbows straight. Give 4 quick, forceful downward and forward thrusts toward the head.

(continued from p. 128)

see if the object appears in the victim's mouth or the top of the throat. Use your fingers to pull the object out.

If the Victim Is Unconscious or Becomes Unconscious:

1. Place the victim on his or her back on a rigid surface, such as the ground.
2. Open the victim's airway by extending the head backward. To do this, place the palm of your hand on the victim's forehead and the fingers of your other hand under the bony part of the chin. Attempt to restore breathing with mouth-to-mouth resuscitation.
3. If still unsuccessful, and with the victim on his or her back, begin the Heimlich maneuver by putting the heel of one hand on the victim's stomach slightly above the navel and below the ribs. Put your free hand on top of your other hand to provide additional force. Keep your elbows straight. Give 4 quick, forceful, downward and forward thrusts toward the head.
4. If these procedures fail, grasp the victim's lower jaw and tongue with one hand and lift up to remove the tongue from the back of the throat. Place the index finger of the other hand inside the victim's mouth alongside the cheek. Slide your fingers down into the throat to the base of the victim's tongue.

   Carefully sweep your fingers along the back of the throat to dislodge the object. Bring your fingers out along the inside of the other cheek. Be careful not to push the object farther down the victim's throat. If a foreign body comes within reach, grasp and

remove it. *Do not* attempt to remove the foreign object with any type of instrument or forceps unless you are trained to do so.
5. Repeat all of the above steps until the object is dislodged or medical assistance arrives. Do not give up!

If the Victim Is an Infant:

1. Place the infant face down across your forearm with his or her head low. Support the head by firmly holding the jaw.
2. Rest your forearm on your thigh. Support the infant's head by firmly holding the jaw. Give 4 forceful back blows with the heel of your hand between the infant's shoulder blades. The blows should be more gentle than those for an adult.
3. If unsuccessful, turn the infant over and give 4 quick thrusts on the chest. To do this, place two fingers one finger-width below an imaginary line joining the nipples. Push downward and forward. Thrusts should be more gentle than those for an adult.
4. If necessary, repeat both procedures.

Heimlich Maneuver on an Infant

Rest your forearm on your thigh. Support the infant's head by firmly holding the jaw. Give 4 forceful back blows with the heel of your hand between the infant's shoulder blades.

If unsuccessful, turn the infant over and give 4 quick thrusts on the chest. To do this, place 2 fingers one finger-width below an imaginary line joining the nipples. Push downward and forward. Thrusts should be more gentle than those for an adult. If necessary, repeat both procedures.

INJURIES AND ILLNESSES

Heimlich Maneuver on a Child

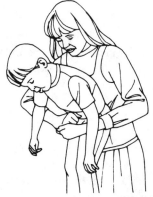

Stand behind the child with your arms around his or her waist. Place the thumb side of your fist against the child's stomach, slightly above the navel and below the ribs and breastbone. Hold your fist with your other hand and give 4 quick, forceful upward thrusts. It may be necessary to repeat the procedure 6 to 10 times.

If the Victim Is Very Fat or Is Pregnant:

Immediate Treatment:

1. Stand behind the victim and place your fist on the middle of the breastbone in the chest, but not over the ribs. Put your other hand on top of it. Give 4 quick, forceful movements. *Do not* squeeze with your arms. Just use your fist.
2. If this procedure does not work, stand behind the victim and support his or her chest with one hand. With the heel of the other hand give 4 quick blows on the back between the victim's shoulder blades.

If You Are Alone and Choking:

Immediate Treatment:

1. Place your fist on your stomach slightly above your navel and below your ribs. Place your other hand on top of it. Give yourself 4 quick, forceful upward abdominal thrusts.
2. If this procedure does not work, press your stomach forcefully over a chair, table, sink, or railing.

See Also: Unconsciousness, p. 251.

CONVULSIONS (SEIZURES)

A convulsion (seizure) results from a disturbance in electrical activity in the brain, causing a series of uncontrollable muscle movements. These may occur during a state of total or partial unconsciousness and there may be a temporary loss of breathing. Most convulsions last 1 to 2 minutes.

Contrary to myth, a person having a seizure is not in danger of biting off his or her tongue. *Do not* put any object into the victim's mouth.

Convulsions may occur with a head injury, brain tumor, epilepsy (see Epileptic Seizure, p. 136), poisoning, electric shock, withdrawal from drugs, heat stroke, scorpion bites, poisonous snake bites, hyperventilation, or high fever—particularly in young children (see Convulsions in Infants and Children, pp. 136–137).

Although convulsions *appear* alarming, they rarely cause serious problems in themselves. Injuries may result from falling during the seizure or from bumping into surrounding objects.

Any or all of the following may be present:

Symptoms
1. The victim utters a short cry or scream.
2. Muscles become rigid, followed by jerky, twitching movements.
3. Breathing may stop temporarily during the seizure.
4. Bluish color appears on the face and lips.
5. Eyes may roll upward.
6. There is possible loss of bladder and bowel control.
7. The victim drools or foams (may be bloody) at the mouth.
8. The victim is unresponsive during the seizure.
9. Sleepiness and confusion overcome the victim after the convulsion is over.

What to Do

1. If the victim starts to fall, try to catch the victim and lay him or her down gently.
2. Remove any surrounding objects that the victim might strike during the convulsion, or remove the victim from dangerous surroundings (such as stairs, glass doors, or a fireplace).
3. If breathing stops and does not start again momentarily after the seizure, maintain an open airway. Check to make sure the victim's tongue is not blocking his or her throat. Restore breathing if necessary after the seizure.

ABCs

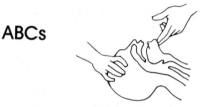

With all serious injuries, check and maintain an open airway. Restore breathing (p. 20) and circulation (p. 22), if necessary.

4. *Do not* interfere with convulsive movements, but be sure that the victim does not injure himself or herself. *Do not* try to hold the victim down, as muscle tears or fractures may result.
5. *Do not* force any object such as a spoon or pencil between the victim's teeth.
6. *Do not* throw any liquid on the victim's face or into his or her mouth.
7. Loosen tight clothing around the victim's neck and waist.
8. After the convulsion is over, turn the victim's head to the side or place the victim on his or her side to prevent choking on secretions, blood, or vomit.
9. Keep the victim lying down after the convulsion is over, as he or she may be confused for a while.
10. If necessary, shield the victim from a crowd to prevent embarrassment.

(continued on p. 136)

Mouth-to-Mouth Resuscitation

If the victim is not breathing and no neck injury is suspected, perform the following 4 steps.

If a neck injury is suspected (as in a diving or motorcycle accident, or from a fall from a height) *do not* twist or rotate the head. *Slightly* elevate the chin only to open the airway. Check for foreign material in the mouth. Then continue with steps 3 and 4, below.*

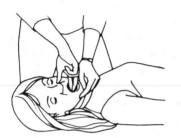

1.) Make sure the victim is on a hard, flat surface. Quickly clear the mouth and airway of foreign material.

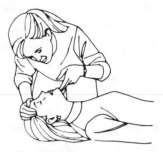

2.) Tilt the victim's head backward by placing the palm of your hand on his or her forehead and the fingers of your other hand under the bony part of the chin.

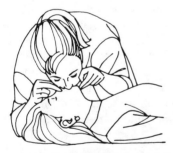

3.) Pinch the victim's nostrils with your thumb and index finger. Take a deep breath. Place your mouth tightly over the victim's mouth (mouth and nose for an infant or small child). Give two quick breaths.

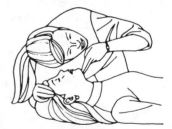

4.) Stop blowing when the chest is expanding. Remove your mouth from the victim's mouth and turn your head toward the victim's chest, so that your ear is over his or her mouth. *Listen* for air being exhaled. *Watch* for the victim's chest to fall. Repeat the breathing procedure.

*To move a victim with a neck injury, see page 191.

11. Check for other injuries, such as bleeding and broken bones, and administer appropriate treatment.
12. Stay with the victim while he or she recovers.
13. Seek medical attention promptly, particularly if the seizure is followed by a second convulsion or if the victim is pregnant.

EPILEPTIC SEIZURE

Epilepsy is a disorder in which the victim usually has a hereditary tendency to have convulsions. It results when certain brain cells temporarily become overactive and release too much electrical energy. Sometimes the victim has a warning sensation (aura) that a seizure is about to occur and often utters a short scream or cry just before the attack. Symptoms during the seizure are the same as those for convulsions (see p. 133).

What to Do The treatment for a known epileptic seizure is the same as for convulsions (see pp. 134–136). The primary aim is to prevent the victim from harming himself or herself. *Do not* interfere with the convulsive movements. After the seizure, maintain an open airway and restore breathing if the victim has stopped breathing and does not start again momentarily. When the seizure is over, allow the victim to rest or sleep. It is always best to consult the victim's doctor. Always seek immediate medical attention if the seizure lasts longer than 5 minutes, if another convulsion follows the first, or if the victim is pregnant.

CONVULSIONS IN INFANTS AND CHILDREN

Convulsions in young children are not uncommon. The most frequent cause is a rapid rise in temperature due to an acute infection.

These convulsions are called febrile convulsions and occur usually in a child between 1 and 4 years of age. Febrile convulsions seldom last longer than 2 to 3 minutes. Although all convulsions in young children must be taken seriously, they are usually more frightening to watch than dangerous. The symptoms for febrile convulsions are the same as for convulsions (see p. 133).

What to Do
1. Do not panic.
2. Maintain an open airway. Check to make sure that the child's tongue is not blocking his or her throat. *If it is, elevate the chin.*

ABCs

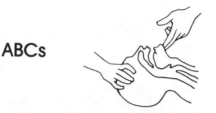

With all serious injuries, check and maintain an open airway. Restore breathing (p. 20) and circulation (p. 22), if necessary.

3. After the seizure, turn the child's head to one side or place the child on his or her side so that he or she will not choke if vomiting should occur.
4. Remove the child's clothes and sponge his or her body with lukewarm water to help reduce the fever.
5. *Do not* place the child in a tub of water as he or she may inhale the water during the convulsion.
6. *Do not* throw water on the child's face or into his or her mouth.
7. Have someone else call the child's doctor during the convulsion if you do not want to leave the child unattended. If this is impossible, call the doctor when the convulsion is over. If the doctor is not available, take the child to the hospital.

See Also: Drug Abuse, p. 154; Fever, p. 177; Headaches, p. 187; Head and Neck Injuries, p. 188; Overexposure: Heat and Cold, p. 209; Poisoning, p. 216; Pregnancy, Danger Signs, p. 221; and Shock, p. 234.

INJURIES AND ILLNESSES

DECOMPRESSION SICKNESS (CAISSON DISEASE)

Also known as the bends, the condition occurs when an individual rises too quickly from a compressed atmosphere (such as very deep water) to a higher altitude. Doing so can cause air bubbles—mostly nitrogen—to form in the blood. An air bubble that travels to the brain can cause instant death (aeroembolism). The sickness occurs in varying degrees of severity *usually* in inexperienced divers and, rarely, in miners.

Symptoms   Any or all of the following may be present:

1. The victim may be bent over with pain.
2. The victim has great difficulty in breathing.
3. Paralysis occurs.
4. There is bleeding from the nose or ears.
5. The victim has pain in the joints.

Immediate   1. Maintain an open airway. Restore breathing
Treatment   and circulation, if necessary.

ABCs

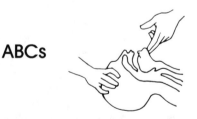

With all serious injuries, check and maintain an open airway. Restore breathing (p. 20) and circulation (p. 22), if necessary.

2. The victim will need immediate medical attention (rapid recompression), preferably at the nearest hospital emergency room.

DEHYDRATION

Dehydration is lack of adequate water in the body. Severe dehydration can occur with vomiting, excessive heat and sweating, diarrhea, or lack of food or fluid intake. Dehydration is a medical emergency and *can be fatal.* The condition is common in the elderly and can occur rapidly in infants and young children.

Symptoms   Any or all of the following may be present:

1. Extreme thirst. The victim may not be able to quench thirst.
2. Tiredness.
3. Lightheadedness.
4. Abdominal or muscle cramping.

What to Do

1. Move the victim into the shade or a cool area.
2. To replace lost fluids and body chemicals, give the victim water, tea, carbonated beverages (shake up to eliminate the fizz), a commercial electrolyte-replacement fluid, flavored gelatin (in liquid form), or clear broth.
3. Seek medical attention if symptoms persist or if other complications (nausea, diarrhea, convulsions) arise.

See Also: Convulsions, p. 133; Diarrhea, p. 144; Overexposure: Heat and Cold (Heat Cramps, Heat Exhaustion, Heatstroke), pp. 209–211; Vomiting, p. 255.

DENTAL EMERGENCIES

TOOTHACHE

Cavities and infections often cause toothaches. Home treatment offers only temporary relief from pain but is often helpful if a toothache occurs in the middle of the night or before you can seek professional attention. A trip to the dentist is necessary to find the exact cause of a toothache and to treat it effectively.

What to Do
1. Give the victim aspirin, acetaminophen, or ibuprofen. Aspirin should be swallowed and not applied directly to the affected area.
2. Place cold compresses or ice packs on the face over the affected area. For some victims, warm compresses may be more comforting. This varies for each individual.
3. Seek dental attention.

KNOCKED-OUT TOOTH (AVULSED TOOTH)

What to Do
1. Treat for bleeding. (See Pulled Tooth, opposite page.)
2. Wrap the tooth in a cool wet cloth or place it in whole milk (not skim milk). Milk has nutrients that will help keep the tooth alive. *Do not* put the tooth in tap water. The minerals in water may cause further harm. Saline (salt) water may be used, however. Take the victim and the tooth to the dentist or hospital emergency room as soon as possible.

PULLED TOOTH (EXTRACTION)

Pain, slight swelling, and bleeding often occur after a tooth has been pulled. If these problems become severe or persistent, consult your dentist.

What to Do
1. As soon as possible after the tooth has been pulled, place a cold compress or ice bag on the face on the affected area to relieve swelling. The compress should remain in place for 15 minutes out of each hour. Repeat the procedure for several hours.
2. If bleeding is present: Fold a clean piece of gauze, handkerchief, or tissue into a pad and place over the wound. Close teeth tightly so that firm pressure is applied against the bleeding area. Maintain pressure for 20 to 30 minutes. Repeat the procedure if necessary.
3. If the dentist did not prescribe medication for pain, aspirin, acetaminophen, or ibuprofen may be taken. Aspirin should be swallowed, *not* placed directly over the wound.

See Also: Head and Neck Injuries, p. 188.

INJURIES AND ILLNESSES

DIABETIC COMA

Diabetic coma occurs when there is too little insulin in the body due to the body's inability to use insulin properly, neglected insulin injections, improper diet, or infections.

ABCs

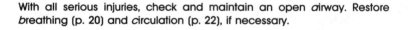

With all serious injuries, check and maintain an open airway. Restore breathing (p. 20) and circulation (p. 22), if necessary.

Symptoms

Symptoms are the opposite of those of insulin shock. Any or all of the following may be present:

1. Gradual onset of symptoms.
2. Extreme thirst.
3. Warm, red, and dry skin.
4. Drowsiness.
5. Fruity-smelling breath.
6. Deep and rapid breathing.
7. Dry mouth and tongue.
8. Nausea, with upper abdominal discomfort.
9. Vomiting.
10. Frequent urination.

Immediate Treatment

Seek medical attention promptly, preferably at the nearest hospital emergency room.

See Also: Unconsciousness, p. 251; Vomiting, p. 255.

Mouth-to-Mouth Resuscitation

If the victim is not breathing and no neck injury is suspected, perform all of the the following 4 steps.

If a neck injury is suspected (as in a diving or motorcycle accident, or from a fall from a height) *do not* twist or rotate the head. *Slightly* elevate the chin only to open the airway. Check for foreign material in the mouth. Then continue with steps 3 and 4, below.*

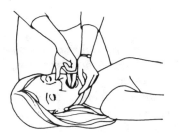

1. Make sure the victim is on a hard, flat surface. Quickly clear the mouth and airway of foreign material.

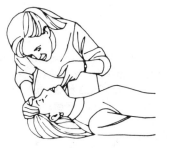

2. Tilt the victim's head backward by placing the palm of your hand on his or her forehead and the fingers of your other hand under the bony part of the chin.

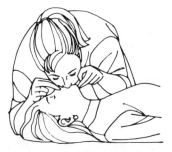

3. Pinch the victim's nostrils with your thumb and index finger. Take a deep breath. Place your mouth tightly over the victim's mouth (mouth and nose for an infant or small child). Give 2 quick breaths.

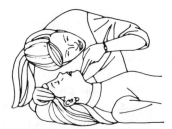

4. Stop blowing when the chest is expanding. Remove your mouth from the victim's mouth and turn your head toward the victim's chest, so that your ear is over his or her mouth. *Listen* for air being exhaled. *Watch* for the victim's chest to fall. Repeat the breathing procedure.

*To move a victim with a neck injury, see p. 191.

DIARRHEA

Diarrhea is frequent elimination or the passage of loose, watery stools. There are many causes of this condition. Among the most common are: food poisoning, mushroom poisoning, dysentery, certain medications, emotional stress, excessive drinking of alcoholic beverages, viral and bacterial infections, and stomach flu (viral gastroenteritis).

If diarrhea is not severe and the individual will take liquids, the body can replace lost fluids. If the individual won't take liquids or is vomiting, replacement of fluids will be impossible and dehydration can occur rapidly. Hospitalization may be necessary.

Adults

Symptoms   Any or all of the following may be present:

1. Frequent loose and watery stools. Stools may vary in color from light tan to green.
2. Stomach cramping.
3. Tiredness (due to loss of potassium).
4. Thirst (due to loss of fluid).
5. Blood streaks in or on stools.

What to Do   1. A liquid diet is recommended to replace lost fluids and some body chemicals. (Drink tea, clear broth, or soup, a commercial electrolyte-replacement drink, a commercially available flavored gelatin (drink it in liquid form), carbonated beverages (shake up to reduce the fizz), or a salt-and-sugar-water solution (see p. 146). Water alone may pass right through.

Drink at least 2 ounces of the solution every hour.

2. If diarrhea persists longer than a day or two, or if urine decreases in both frequency and amount, seek medical attention because fatal dehydration may occur.

3. *Avoid* solid foods.

WARNING: If symptoms continue and if bloody stools or stools that are black in color occur or if severe or prolonged stomach cramping occurs, seek prompt medical attention at your doctor's office or hospital emergency room.

Infants and Children

Common causes of diarrhea in infants and children are infection, spoiled food, food allergies or intolerance, foods with laxative effects, and poisoning.

If diarrhea is not severe and the child will take liquids, the body can replace lost fluids. If the child won't take liquids or is vomiting, replacement of fluids will be impossible and dehydration can occur rapidly, *especially in infants and children.* Hospitalization may be necessary.

Symptoms   Frequent elimination of loose, watery stools. (Stools may or may not have a bad odor.)

What to Do   1. A liquid diet is recommended to replace lost fluids and some body chemicals. (Have the infant or child drink a clear broth or soup, apple juice, a commercial electrolyte-replacement drink, a commercially available flavored gelatin (prepare it to drink in liquid form), carbonated beverages (shake up to eliminate the fizz), or a salt-and-sugar-water solution. (See p. 146.) Water alone may pass right through the infant or child. Have him or her drink at least 2 ounces every hour.

2. *Avoid* solid foods.

WARNING: Diarrhea in infants can rapidly lead to severe dehydration or may indicate other serious problems.

INJURIES AND ILLNESSES

If the following danger signals occur, seek medical attention promptly:

1. Three or four loose, watery stools, every 4 to 6 hours.
2. Fever.
3. Dry mouth.
4. Decreased urination in both frequency and amount.
5. Drowsiness, sluggishness, weak cry.
6. Sunken eyes.
7. Vomiting.
8. Blood in the stools.

Salt-and-Sugar-Water Solution

1 quart of water
1 teaspoon of salt
1 tablespoon of sugar
4 teaspoons cream of tartar
½ teaspoon of baking soda

Mix the ingredients together and drink at least 2 ounces every hour. If cream of tartar and baking soda are not available, use just the water, salt, and sugar.

See Also: Abdominal Pain, p. 53; Food Poisoning, p. 183; Vomiting, p. 255.

DISLOCATIONS

A dislocation occurs when the end of a bone is displaced from its joint. It usually results from a fall or a blow to the bone. Common areas of dislocations include the shoulder, hip, elbow, fingers, thumb, and kneecap.

Symptoms   Any or all of the following may be present:

1. Swelling.
2. Deformity at the joint.
3. Pain upon attempting to move the injured part or inability to move the part.
4. Discoloration of the skin around the area of the injury.
5. Tenderness upon touching the area.

What to Do   1. *Do not* try to put a dislocated bone back into its place. Unskilled handling can cause extensive damage to nerves and blood vessels. The bone may also be fractured and any movement may cause further tissue damage.
2. Place the victim in a comfortable position.
3. Immobilize the injured part with a splint, pillow, or sling, in the position in which it was found. (See Splinting and Other Procedures, pp. 95–107.)
4. Seek medical attention promptly, preferably at the nearest hospital emergency room.

See Also: Broken Bones and Spinal Injuries, p. 93; Sprains, p. 243; Wounds, p. 257; and Part III: Sports First Aid (pp. 265–319).

INJURIES AND ILLNESSES

DROWNING

In all emergencies involving a drowning person, remember first to be careful of your own safety. In deep water, a drowning person can drag a rescuer under water. Keep calm and do not overestimate your strength. If another person is with you, have that person call for help.

People who have been submerged in cold water (below 70° F) often can survive without brain damage. Some victims have been submerged for as long as 38 minutes and have lived. A reflex most prominent in young children slows the heartbeat and reserves the oxygen in the blood for the heart and brain. Mouth-to-mouth breathing and CPR must be started as soon as possible and continued, *often for several hours,* until the victim's body has become warm and he or she begins breathing on his or her own. Further medical treatment at a doctor's office or hospital emergency room will also be necessary.

How to
Rescue
from Water

If a drowning victim is near a pier or the side of a swimming pool, lie down and give the victim your hand or foot and pull him or her to safety. If the victim is too far away, hold out a life preserver ring, pole, stick, board, rope, chair, tree limb, towel, or other object.

If the victim is out from the shore, wade into the water and extend a pole, board, stick, or rope to the victim and pull him or her to safety. It may be necessary to row a boat to the victim. If so, hand the victim an oar or other suitable object and pull him or her to the boat. If possible, the victim

A Rescue from Water

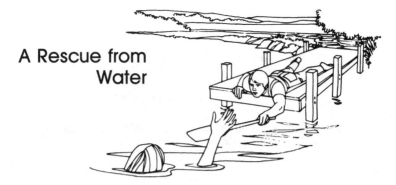

If a drowning victim is near a pier, but too far away to reach your hand or foot, lie down and hold out a pole, paddle, or life preserver, and pull the victim to safety.

should hold on to the back of the boat while being rowed to the shore. If this is not possible, pull the victim carefully into the boat.

If a Neck or Back Injury Is Suspected (from a Diving or Surfboard Accident):

What to Do   If trained medical personnel are not available to assist you, place a board (surfboard, table leaf) under the victim's head and back while he or she is still in the water. (The board should extend from the head to the buttocks.) This will keep the victim from moving, thus preventing further damage to the neck or back. Lift the victim out of the water on the board.

*If the Victim Is **Not** Breathing:*

Immediate   Artificial breathing must be started *at once,* before
Treatment   the victim is completely out of the water, if possible. As soon as the victim's body can be supported, either in a boat or in shallow water, start mouth-to-mouth breathing. (See p. 20.) Once the victim is out of the water, lay him or her on the back on a firm surface and continue mouth-to-mouth resuscitation and CPR if necessary. (See p. 22.)

Do not waste time trying to drain water from the victim's lungs.

ABCs

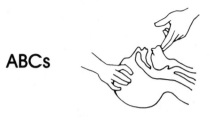

With all serious injuries, check and maintain an open *airway*. Restore *breathing* (p. 20) and *circulation* (p. 22), if necessary.

If a Board Is Not Available:

What to Do   Gently tow or push the victim to shallow water and stay with him or her. *Do not* drag the victim sideways. Pull him or her by the armpits or legs in the direction of the length of the body. Keep the head in line with the body. Call for help or have someone get help for you.

      If the victim is face down in the water, gently turn him or her over, keeping the head, neck, and body in alignment.

NOTE: *It is inadvisable to move a victim with a suspected neck injury unless the victim's life and yours are in danger.*

    Remember that *any* movement of the head, either forward, backward, or side to side, can result in paralysis or death.

    If you must move the victim, *always keep the head, neck, and body in alignment.* (See p. 99 and p. 191.)

(*continued on p. 152*)

Mouth-to-Mouth Resuscitation

If the victim is not breathing and no neck injury is suspected, perform all of the following 4 steps.

If a neck injury is suspected (as in a diving accident), *do not* twist or rotate the head. *Slightly* elevate the chin only to open the airway. Check for foreign material in the mouth. Then continue with steps 3 and 4, below.*

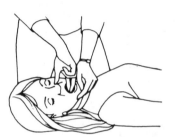

1. Make sure the victim is on a hard, flat surface. Quickly clear the mouth and airway of foreign material.

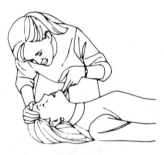

2. Tilt the victim's head backward by placing the palm of your hand on his or her forehead and the fingers of your other hand under the bony part of the chin.

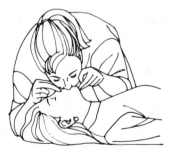

3. Pinch the victim's nostrils with your thumb and index finger. Take a deep breath. Place your mouth tightly over the victim's mouth (mouth and nose for an infant or small child). Give 2 quick breaths.

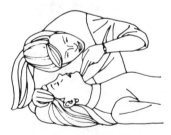

4. Stop blowing when the chest is expanding. Remove your mouth from the victim's mouth and turn your head toward the victim's chest, so that your ear is over his or her mouth. *Listen* for air being exhaled. *Watch* for the victim's chest to fall. Repeat the breathing procedure.

*To move a victim with a neck injury, see p. 191.

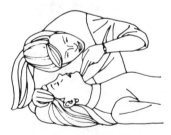

(continued from p. 150)
If the Victim Is Breathing:

Immediate
Treatment

1. Watch the victim to ensure that he or she continues to breathe on his or her own.
2. Place the victim on his or her side with head extended backward so that fluids will drain.
3. Keep the victim comfortably warm.
4. Reassure the victim.
5. Watch for signs of shock. (See Shock, p. 234.)
6. Seek medical attention promptly. *Do not* give the victim food or water.

To Aid a Drowning Victim

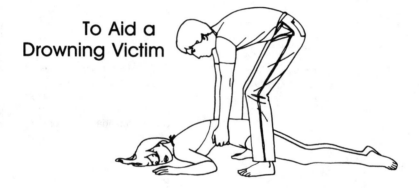

To remove water from a victim's stomach, place both hands under the stomach and lift.

SHALLOW WATER BLACKOUT

The condition occurs when an individual—usually a child—hyperventilates on purpose in an effort to stay under water for a longer period of time. The process of hyperventilation, however, removes carbon dioxide from the blood, which at normal levels triggers the involuntary stimulus to breathe. While the individual can actually stay longer under water, he or she may pass out due to the lack of oxygen. If not caught in time, the individual may drown.

Symptoms   1. The victim has been under water, or face down
                in the water, longer than usual.
            2. The victim appears lifeless in the water.

ABCs

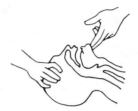

With all serious injuries, check and maintain an open airway. Restore
breathing (p. 20) and circulation (p. 22), if necessary.

Immediate   1. Remove the victim at once from the water.
Treatment   2. Maintain an open airway. Restore breathing
                and circulation if necessary, p. 20.
            3. Take the victim to the nearest hospital emer-
                gency room for further evaluation.

See Also: Head and Neck Injuries, pp. 188–195.

INJURIES AND ILLNESSES

DRUG ABUSE

Drug abuse is the regular or excessive use of a drug outside the usual standards of medical practice or medical need. Drug abuse often results in physical and psychological dependence on the drug.*

Questions to ask yourself if you suspect that someone you know is using drugs are: How is the individual acting *different from normal*? Is he or she overly quiet, moody, or easily agitated? Are there physical manifestations that might warn one of drug use, such as a sudden loss of weight or an inattention to personal hygiene? Has the individual's group of friends changed within the past six months? Do you know who they are? Or, alternatively, has the person stopped seeing his or her friends? Does he or she spend more time alone?

Mild changes in behavior, especially in teenagers, do not necessarily mean that an individual is taking drugs. If you suspect drug use, however, other clues may be helpful in identifying the problem.

Clues to Look For	Use of any drug either depresses the central nervous system or activates it. Depending upon the type and the amount of the drug taken, a person's behavior under the influence of that drug may range from extreme sluggishness to hyperactivity. With drugs that are injected into the body, you may notice needle marks on the victim's arms or legs (or elsewhere). In cases of drug withdrawal, you may notice frequent blinking or jerky eye

---

*If you are using drugs, this section will provide you with information about drug overdose and withdrawal and first-aid measures for yourself or for another person. We strongly urge that you see a physician for a confidential discussion about your drug habits and for information concerning immediate treatment.

movements in the victim, along with other symptoms listed on the following pages.

Paraphernalia that may signal drug use include needles, eye droppers, teaspoons, pills, capsules, vials, pipes, glass bulbs ("bongs"), or other drug containers you may not be familiar with.

Immediate Treatment

1. Professional medical treatment for a person who is suffering withdrawal from drugs or who has overdosed on drugs will vary according to the type and amount of the drug taken.
2. For the first-aider faced with an emergency situation in which drug use is suspected, first assess whether or not it is safe for you to handle the situation on your own. If it is not, call out for help.
3. If the victim is unconscious, ensure that he or she is breathing. Restore breathing and circulation, if necessary.

ABCs

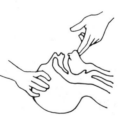

With all serious injuries, check and maintain an open airway. Restore breathing (p. 20) and circulation (p. 22), if necessary.

4. If the victim is conscious and you are the first person providing first aid, ask the victim what drug he or she took, the amount, and when it was taken. (Report all information, including first-aid treatment, to the doctor assuming care of the victim.)
5. The victim, under the influence of a drug, may try to harm you. If the victim is seen taking a drug by mouth and is alert, cooperative, and in good control of himself or herself, induce vomiting by tickling or touching the back of the

INJURIES AND ILLNESSES

victim's throat with your finger. Take care that
the victim does not choke on the vomit.

Additional information about drug overdose and withdrawal, by
category of drug, is given on the following pages.

ALCOHOL

Ethanol is the active or "toxic" ingredient in all alcoholic beverages
that causes intoxication. It slows down or depresses the activities of
the central nervous system (the brain and spinal cord) that control
psychomotor skills, such as reaction time and coordination, and
other areas of the brain that control speech, hearing, and eye movement. Alcohol also impairs reasoning by relaxing an individual's
social inhibitions and conscious self-control.

Ingesting alcoholic beverages can give a false sense of euphoria.
Alcohol can appear to act as a stimulant but, in fact, is a depressant.

Alcoholic beverages include beer, light beer, wine, wine coolers,
hard liquor, and "spirits," such as cognac, sherry, and other after-
dinner drinks.

Overdose

Symptoms   Any or all of the following may be present:

1. Lack of coordination.
2. Slurred speech.
3. Abnormal breathing.
4. Unconsciousness.
5. Possible coma.
6. Red streaks in the whites
   of the eyes.
7. Odor of alcohol.

Immediate
Treatment
1. If the victim appears to be sleeping, with normal breathing and pulse, and he or she can be
   aroused with a shout or a shake, no immediate
   treatment is required. Place the victim so that
   he or she will not hurt himself or herself.
   Check on the victim at regular intervals.
2. If the victim has abnormal breathing, is unconscious (cannot be aroused), or is in a coma,
   maintain an open airway. Restore breathing
   and circulation, if necessary.
3. Seek medical attention promptly.

ABCs

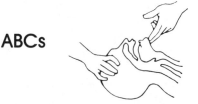

With all serious injuries, check and maintain an open airway. Restore breathing (p. 20) and circulation (p. 22), if necessary.

Withdrawal

Symptoms   Any or all of the following may be present:

1. Trembling of hands and head.
2. Nausea.
3. Vomiting.
4. Fear of sounds, ordinary objects, or lights.
5. Possible hallucinations (seeing or hearing objects that are not present).
6. Other unusual behavior.
7. High fever.

Immediate   1. Maintain an open airway. Restore breathing
Treatment   and circulation, if necessary.
2. If the victim is vomiting, see that he or she does not choke on vomit.
3. Calm and reassure the victim.
4. Seek medical attention promptly.

DEPRESSANTS

Depressants slow down or depress the activities of the central nervous system (the brain and spinal cord) that control psychomotor skills, such as reaction time and coordination, and other functions of the brain that control speech, hearing, eye movement, and perception.

Depressants include all alcoholic beverages (see p. 156), narcotics, sedatives, cannabis drugs, and all depressant tranquilizers. Examples are opium, morphine, heroin, Fentanyl (synthetic heroin), codeine, downers, phenobarbital, "goofballs," "yellow jackets," "red devils," "rainbows," sleeping pills, marijuana, and hashish.

Overdose

Symptoms   Any or all of the following may be present:

1. Drunklike behavior.
2. Slurred speech.
3. Sleep, possibly leading to coma.
4. Shallow breathing.

5. Slow pulse.
6. Low body temperature.
7. Heavy sweating.
8. Very relaxed muscles.
9. Very small eye pupils.

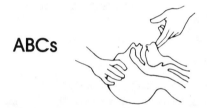

ABCs

With all serious injuries, check and maintain an open airway. Restore breathing (p. 20) and circulation (p. 22), if necessary.

Immediate
Treatment

1. Maintain an open airway. Restore breathing and circulation, if necessary.
2. Keep the victim awake. Using a cold, wet towel or cloth, slap the victim's face gently.
3. Keep the victim talking, if possible.
4. Calm and reassure the victim.
5. Seek medical attention promptly.

Withdrawal

Symptoms   Any or all of the following may be present:

1. Nervousness, restlessness.
2. Trembling.
3. Muscle twitching.
4. Abdominal cramping.
5. Hot and cold flashes.
6. Sweating.

7. Tears.
8. Runny nose.
9. Yawning.
10. Muscle aches.
11. Vomiting.
12. Loss of appetite.

13.	Weight loss.	15.	Rise in body temperature.
14.	Enlarged eye pupils.	16.	Craving for the drug.

Symptoms may not occur all at the same time.

ABCs

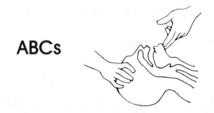

With all serious injuries, check and maintain an open *airway*. Restore *breathing* (p. 20) and *circulation* (p. 22), if necessary.

Immediate Treatment
1. Maintain an open airway. Restore breathing and circulation, if necessary.
2. Calm and reassure the victim.
3. Seek medical attention if the discomfort is severe.

HALLUCINOGENS

Hallucinogenic drugs, also called psychedelic drugs, alter perceptions of reality. They change the chemical makeup of the brain.

Hallucinogenic drugs include: LSD, PCP, mescaline (peyote buttons), and psilocybin (mushrooms). Amphetamines, other stimulants, and THC, the active ingredient in marijuana and hashish, can also be hallucinogenic.

Overdose

Symptoms   Any or all of the following may be present:

1. Delusions (misinterpretation of sounds, movements, or objects).
2. Hallucinations, visions (seeing things or hearing sounds that have no factual basis).
3. Fast heartbeat.
4. Increased blood pressure.

INJURIES AND ILLNESSES

5. Enlarged eye pupils.
6. Reddish face.
7. Lack of emotional control (periods of laughing and crying; behavior not appropriate for the situation or the questions asked).
8. Depression (appearing sad; slow to move or talk).
9. Panic, fear, tension.
10. Varying levels of consciousness.
11. Disorientation.
12. Poor recent memory.

Immediate Treatment

1. Ensure that the victim does not harm himself or herself or others.
2. Reassure the victim and try to talk him or her through the experience while in a quiet and peaceful place.
3. Do not move suddenly in front of the victim. Keep your voice calm and do not turn away from the victim. The victim, under the influence of a drug, may try to harm you.
4. Seek medical attention promptly.

STIMULANTS

Stimulants increase or stimulate the activities of the central nervous system (brain and spinal cord) that control psychomotor skills, such as reaction time and coordination, and other areas of the brain that control speech, hearing, eye movement, and perception.

These drugs include all stimulants, inhalants, and antidepressant tranquilizers. Examples include cocaine, "crack," "ice" ("crystal meth"), "speed," "uppers," "pep pills," "bennies," "whites," "dexies," glue, paints and lacquers and their thinners, gasoline, kerosene, nail polish and remover, and lighter fluid.

Overdose

Symptoms Any or all of the following may be present:

1. Overly active behavior.
2. Aggressive behavior.
3. Mental confusion.
4. Disorganization.
5. Repetition of a particular act over and over.
6. Irritableness.
7. Fear.

8. Suspiciousness.

9. Exaggerated perceptions of personal abilities.

ABCs

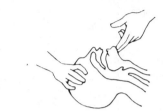

With all serious injuries, check and maintain an open *airway*. Restore *breathing* (p. 20) and *circulation* (p. 22), if necessary.

Immediate Treatment
1. Approach the victim carefully.
2. Maintain an open airway. Restore breathing and circulation, if necessary.
3. Seek medical attention.
4. Keep victim from harming himself or others.

Withdrawal

Symptoms   Any or all of the following may be present:

1. Extreme lack of energy.
2. Depression.
3. Extreme hunger.

4. Hallucinations.
5. Deep sleep.
6. Dehydration.

ABCs

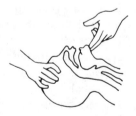

With all serious injuries, check and maintain an open *airway*. Restore *breathing* (p. 20) and *circulation* (p. 22), if necessary.

Immediate Treatment
1. Maintain an open airway. Restore breathing and circulation, if necessary.
2. Seek medical attention if symptoms are severe.

EAR INJURIES AND EARACHES

BLEEDING FROM THE EAR

A ruptured eardrum can be caused by a loud blast, by an infection, by diving into water, by falls from waterskiing, by objects poked into the ear, or as a result of a head injury. Blood or other fluids coming from the ear canal may mean a serious head injury.

Symptoms   Any or all of the following may be present:

1. Bleeding from inside the ear canal.
2. Pain.
3. Hearing loss.

Immediate   1. If bleeding is due to a head injury with a possi-
Treatment   ble skull fracture, treat the head injury first. (See Head and Neck Injuries, pp. 188–195.)
2. *Do not* put anything into the ear.
3. *Do not* try to stop the flow of blood from the ear canal.
4. Loosely cover the outside of the ear with a bandage or cloth to catch the flow of blood.
5. Place the victim on his or her injured side so that the affected ear is downward, allowing blood to drain. The victim should not be moved if a serious neck, head, or back injury is suspected unless his or her life is in jeopardy.
6. Seek medical attention promptly.

EARACHES

There are many causes for pain in the ear. One of the most common is an infection of the outer ear caused by a scratch, as from a fingernail, or by swimming in contaminated water, which can cause "swimmer's ear."

Symptoms of "swimmer's ear" may include pain (particularly when the ear is pulled), itching, and a discharge from the ear. This condition requires medical attention.

Occasionally, one will feel ear pain that is caused by a medical problem elsewhere in the body, such as a sore throat or temporomandibular joint syndrome (TMJ), in which the ligaments, muscles, and joints of the jaw are out of alignment.

Earaches in the middle ear often follow respiratory infections. Germs in the nose and throat move through the Eustachian tube to the middle ear. Children are particularly subject to middle ear infections because their Eustachian tubes are shorter than those of adults. Infected tonsils may also cause a middle ear infection. Symptoms of middle ear infection may include pain, fever, and, rarely, a discharge from the ear. An infant with an ear infection cries loudly, particularly when lying down, pulls or bats at his or her ear, or turns his or her head from side to side.

Medical attention is required for treatment of middle ear infections.

NOTE: Do not *put cotton-tipped swabs, hairpins, matches, or anything else in the ear.*

FOREIGN OBJECTS INSIDE THE EAR

Children often put objects into their ears. The most common objects are peas, beans, beads, paper, and cotton. Insects may also get trapped inside the ear.

What to Do   1.   If an insect inside the ear is alive and buzzing, put several drops of warm oil (baby, mineral, or olive oil) into the ear to kill the insect. This is the only time putting oil into the ear is justified. Seek medical attention for removal of the insect.

2. Other small objects trapped inside the ear need medical attention for removal. The only possible exception is paper or cotton *if* it is *clearly* visible outside the ear canal. In this instance, you may attempt to remove the object carefully with tweezers. A doctor should be seen, however, to make sure all of it is removed.

3. *Do not* put water or oil into the ears to attempt to flush out the object. This may cause the object to swell and make removal more difficult.

FROSTBITE

Symptoms   Any or all of the following may be present:

1. In the earliest stages the skin appears red. Pain is often present.
2. As frostbite develops, the skin becomes white or grayish yellow and appears waxy.
3. Ears feel very cold and numb.
4. Pain disappears.
5. Blisters may occur.
6. Often the victim is not aware that he or she has frostbite until someone else notices the symptoms.

Immediate Treatment

1. While outside, cover the ears with extra clothing or a warm cloth.
2. *Do not* rub the ears with snow or anything else.
3. Bring the victim inside promptly.
4. Frostbitten ears must be rewarmed rapidly. Gently wrap the ears in warm materials, such as moist, warm compresses or dry towels heated in an oven to 100–103°F. Or place the palms of your hands over the victim's ears.
5. *Do not* use heat lamps, hot water bottles, or heating pads.
6. *Do not* allow the victim to place frostbitten ears near a hot stove or radiator. Frostbitten parts may become burned before feeling returns.

7. *Do not* break the blisters. Blisters are a natural barrier against infection.
8. Stop the rewarming process when the skin becomes pink.
9. Seek medical attention promptly.

Continued Care

1. Give the victim warm drinks such as tea, coffee, or soup.
2. Do not give the victim alcoholic beverages. (Alcohol restricts the blood flow.)
3. Take extreme care that frostbitten ears are not refrozen after they have thawed.

Danger Signals

If severe frostbite has occurred, the victim may not have feeling in his or her ears and the ears may be black in color, meaning that the skin tissue has died.

WARNING: If severe frostbite has occurred, cover the ears with warm materials and take the victim *without delay* to the nearest hospital emergency room for treatment.

See Also: Head and Neck Injuries, p. 188.

INJURIES AND ILLNESSES

ELECTRIC SHOCK

WARNING: If you are the first person offering first aid:

It is extremely important to remain calm. *Do not* touch the victim directly until the electric current is turned off or the victim is no longer in contact with it. Otherwise, you risk electrocution yourself. Victims who have been struck by lightning, however, may be touched immediately because they are no longer connected to continuous electricity.

What to Do   1.   If possible, turn off the electric current by removing the fuse or by pulling the main switch.

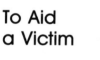

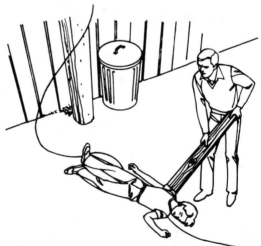

Be extremely careful when removing the victim from a live wire. Stand on a *dry* area.. Push the victim away from the wire with a *dry* board or other *dry* object. *Never* use anything metallic or wet. *Do not* touch the victim until he or she is free from the wire.

If this is not possible, or if the victim is outside, have someone call the electric company to cut off the electricity.

2. If it is necessary to remove the victim from a live wire, be extremely careful. Stand on something *dry,* such as a newspaper, board, blanket, rubber mat, or cloth, and, if possible, wear *dry* gloves.

3. Push the victim away from the wire with a *dry* board, stick, or broom handle, or pull the victim away with a *dry* rope looped around the victim's arm or leg. *Never* use anything metallic, wet, or damp. Do not touch the victim until he or she is free from the wire.

If the victim is not breathing:

Immediate Treatment

1. Maintain an open airway. Restore breathing and circulation, if necessary.

ABCs

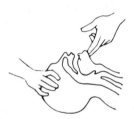

With all serious injuries, check and maintain an open airway. Restore breathing (p. 20) and circulation (p. 22), if necessary.

Mouth-to-Mouth Resuscitation

If the victim is not breathing and no neck injury is suspected, perform all of the following 4 steps.

If a neck injury is suspected (as in a diving or motorcycle accident, or from a fall from a height) *do not* twist or rotate the head. *Slightly* elevate the chin only to open the airway. Check for foreign material in the mouth. Then continue with steps 3 and 4, below.*

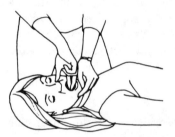

1. Make sure the victim is on a hard, flat surface. Quickly clear the mouth and airway of foreign material.

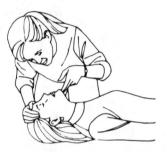

2. Tilt the victim's head backward by placing the palm of your hand on his or her forehead and the fingers of your other hand under the bony part of the chin.

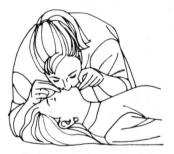

3. Pinch the victim's nostrils with your thumb and index finger. Take a deep breath. Place your mouth tightly over the victim's mouth (mouth and nose for an infant or small child). Give 2 quick breaths.

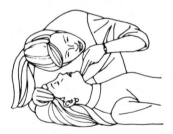

4. Stop blowing when the chest is expanding. Remove your mouth from the victim's mouth and turn your head toward the victim's chest, so that your ear is over his or her mouth. *Listen* for air being exhaled. *Watch* for the victim's chest to fall. Repeat the breathing procedure.

*To move a victim with a neck injury, see p. 191.

EYE INJURIES

CHEMICAL BURNS

Acids, drain cleaner, bleach, and other cleaning solutions are some chemical agents that can burn the eye.

WARNING: Chemical burns of the eye are very serious and may lead to blindness if immediate action is not taken. Speed in removing a chemical agent is vital. Damage can occur in 1 to 5 minutes.

Immediate
Treatment

1. *Before* calling a doctor, immediately flush the eye with large quantities of cool, running water for at least 10 minutes to rinse out the offending agent. Use milk if water is not available. Hold the victim's head under a faucet (or use a glass of water), with the eyelids held open, and allow the water to run from the inside corner (next to the nose) outward so that the water flows over the entire eye and so that the chemical does not get in the unaffected eye. If both eyes are affected, let water flow over both or quickly alternate from one eye to the other. Be sure to lift and separate eyelids so that all parts of the eye will be reached by the water.

2. Another method is to place the top of the victim's face in a bowl or sink filled with water with the eyes in the water, and have the victim move the eyelids up and down.

3. If the victim is lying down, pour large quantities of water from a container from the inside

corner of the eye outward, keeping the eyelids open. Keep repeating this procedure.

4. After following the above steps, cover the injured eye or eyes with a pad of sterile gauze or a clean folded handkerchief, and bandage in place. Eyelids should be closed.

To Flush Out the Eye

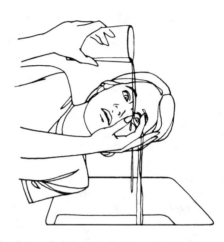

Before calling a doctor, immediately flush the eye with large quantities of cool running water for at least 10 minutes. Allow the water to run from the inside corner outward. Lift and separate the eyelids so that all parts of the eye will be covered by the water.

5. *Do not* allow the victim to rub the eyes.
6. Seek medical attention immediately, preferably at the nearest hospital emergency room.

BLUNT INJURIES (BLACK EYE)

Any injury resulting from a hard direct blow to the eye, such as from a moving ball or a fist, needs medical attention by an ophthalmologist even though the injury may not look serious. There may be internal bleeding in the eye.

Immediate Treatment

1. Apply *cold* compresses to the injured eye.
2. If possible, keep the victim lying down with eyes closed.
3. Seek medical attention.

COMMON EYE INFECTIONS

Chalazion

A chalazion is an infection and inflammation of a deep gland in the eyelid.

Symptoms   1. A hard, red, painful bump in the underside of the eyelid.

What to Do   1. Apply warm water compresses to the outer eyelid several times a day.
2. Do not try to "pop" the bump.
3. If the bump persists longer than several days or recurs, seek medical attention.

Pinkeye (Conjunctivitis)

Pinkeye is an infection of the eye that is usually caused by a fungus, bacteria, allergies, or chemicals. It may affect one or both eyes. Certain forms of pinkeye are very contagious.

Symptoms   1. Redness of the white portion of the eye.
2. Watery or sticky discharge (colored yellow, green, or brown) from the eye.
3. Possible sticking together of the upper and lower eyelashes, particularly when the victim rises in the morning.
4. Sensation of something in the eye.

What to Do   1. Consult a physician.
2. Place an ice cube in a plastic bag and hold over the eyelid. This offers *temporary* relief of pain.
3. Wash your hands (and towels and face cloths) after any contact with the infected eye.

Stye

A stye is an inflammation of the glands of the edge of the eyelid.

Symptoms   1. Tender, red bumps near the edge of the eyelid.
2. Itching or tearing.

What to Do
1. Apply warm water compresses to the affected area several times a day.
2. *Do not* try to "pop" this pimplelike bump or bumps.
3. If the stye persists longer than several days or recurs, seek medical attention.

NOTE: *Any sudden pain in the eyes without recent injury, or a sudden blurring or loss of vision, requires immediate medical attention.*

CONTACT LENSES

In eye injuries in which the victim is wearing contact lenses, the lenses should be removed by a physician as soon as possible.

CUTS

Any cuts to the eye, including the eyelid, can be very serious and could lead to blindness if immediate action is not taken.

Immediate Treatment
1. Cover the injured eye with a sterile pad or gauze or a clean folded cloth and bandage in place, but apply no pressure. Also cover the other uninjured eye to prevent eyeball movement.
2. Seek medical attention immediately, preferably from a physician who is an eye specialist (such as an ophthalmologist) or at the nearest hospital emergency room. Transport the victim lying down flat on his or her back if possible.

FOREIGN BODIES IN THE EYE

WARNING: *Never* attempt to remove any particle that is sticking into the eyeball. Seek immediate medical attention for such injuries. See Immediate Treatment, which follows.

Particles such as eyelashes, cinders, or specks that are resting or floating on the eyeball or inside the eyelid may be carefully removed.

Symptoms	1.	Pain.
	2.	Burning sensation.
	3.	Tearing.
	4.	Redness of the eye.
	5.	Sensitivity to light.

If the Foreign Body Is Sticking into *the Eyeball:*

Immediate
Treatment

1. *Do not* allow the victim to rub his or her eyes.
2. Wash your hands with soap and water before carefully examining the victim's eyes.
3. If the foreign body is sticking into the eyeball, *do not* attempt to remove it.
4. Gently cover *both* eyes (because when one moves, so does the other) with sterile or clean compresses and bandage lightly in place around the victim's head. If compresses are not available, use a scarf, a large cloth napkin, or other suitable material and tie around the victim's head.
5. Seek medical attention promptly, preferably from an eye specialist or at the nearest hospital emergency room. Keep the victim lying down on his or her back while riding to the hospital. Use a stretcher if possible.

If the Foreign Body Is Resting *or* Floating on *the Eyeball or Inside the Eyelid:*

What to Do

1. *Do not* allow the victim to rub his or her eyes.
2. Wash your hands with soap and water before carefully examining the victim's eyes.
3. Gently pull the upper eyelid down over the lower eyelid and hold for a moment. This causes tears to flow, which may wash out the particle.
4. If the particle has not been removed, fill a medicine dropper with warm water and squeeze water over the eye to flush out the particle. If a medicine dropper is not available, hold the victim's head under a gentle stream of running water, or use a glass of water, to flush out the particle.

INJURIES AND ILLNESSES

5. If still unsuccessful, gently pull the lower eye-
    lid down. If the foreign body can be seen on the
    inside of the lower lid, carefully lift the particle
    out with a moistened corner of a clean hand-
    kerchief, cloth, or facial tissue.

To Remove a Particle

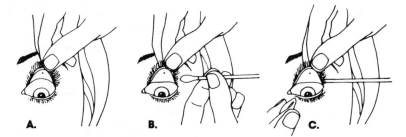

A. Note the particle resting on the inside of the upper lid. The victim must
   look downward during the procedure to remove the particle. Hold
   lashes of the upper eyelid and pull downward.
B. While holding the eyelid down, place a kitchen match or the end of a
   cotton-tipped swab horizontally across the back of the lid and flip the
   eyelid backward over the stick.
C. Carefully remove the particle with the moistened corner of a handkerchief, cloth, or facial tissue.

6. If the speck is not visible on the lower lid,
    check the inside of the upper lid. This can be
    done by first holding the lashes of the upper
    eyelid and pulling downward. The victim must
    look downward during the entire procedure.
    While holding the eyelid down, place a kitchen
    match or the end of a cotton-tipped swab hori-
    zontally across the back of the lid and flip the
    eyelid backward over the stick. (The victim
    can help by holding the stick.) Carefully re-
    move the particle with the moistened corner of
    a handkerchief, cloth, or facial tissue.
7. If the particle still remains, gently cover the
    eye with a sterile or clean compress.
8. Seek medical attention promptly.

See Also: Head and Neck Injuries, p. 188.

FAINTING

Fainting is a brief loss of consciousness due to a reduced blood supply reaching the brain. Recovery usually occurs within a few minutes.

ABCs

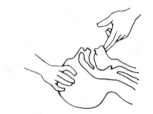

With all serious injuries, check and maintain an open *airway*. Restore *breathing* (p. 20) and *circulation* (p. 22), if necessary.

Symptoms   Any or all of the following may be present:

1. Pale, cool, and wet skin.
2. Lightheadedness.
3. Nausea.

Symptoms may precede or occur during fainting.

To Prevent Fainting:

What to Do   1. Have the victim lie down with legs elevated 8 to 12 inches, or have the victim sit down and slowly bend the body forward so that his or her head is between the knees.
2. Move any harmful objects out of the victim's way.
3. Calm and reassure the victim.

If Fainting Has Occurred:

**Immediate
Treatment**

1. Keep the victim lying down. Elevate the victim's feet 8 to 12 inches from the floor unless a head injury is suspected (from falling).
2. Maintain an open airway.
3. Loosen tight clothing, particularly around the victim's neck.
4. If the victim vomits, place him or her on his or her side. Or, turn the head sideways to prevent choking on vomit.
5. Gently bathe the victim's face with cool water. *Do not* pour water on the victim's face.
6. Check body parts for swelling or deformity that may have been caused by falling.
7. *Do not* give the victim anything to drink unless he or she seems fully recovered.
8. Observe the victim after he or she regains consciousness. Calm and reassure the victim.
9. If recovery does not seem complete within a few minutes, seek medical attention.

FEVER

A fever is the body's way of indicating that something is wrong within it. Most commonly, a fever indicates that an infection is present. It is the body's defensive mechanism to combat infection.

A doctor should always be called if a fever suddenly changes from slight (99°F to 100°F) to high (104°F) and persists. If the victim is an infant and the doctor cannot be reached, take the infant to the nearest hospital emergency room. The same steps should be taken if a fever is present for no obvious reason and it persists. (It is best not to take any medication to reduce the fever in this case, as this may give a false sense of well-being and discourage you from consulting a doctor.)

ADULTS

The average normal temperature taken by mouth is 98.6°F (37°C), plus or minus 1°. A rectal temperature is 1° higher than a normal oral temperature. Individual normal temperatures may run slightly above or below the average. Individual temperatures may also vary throughout the day, running lower in the morning and higher in the evening. Slight changes in temperature (other than normal variations during the day) are usually not significant. A major increase in temperature (to approximately 104°F or over) may indicate a serious condition. However, temperatures well below normal may also be significant. (See Overexposure: Heat and Cold, p. 209.)

What to Do   Aspirin, ibuprofen, and acetaminophen are helpful in reducing a fever. Also, remove excessive clothing and remove the victim from an unusually warm

environment. Follow the package recommendations or a doctor's instructions in determining the
dosage of aspirin to be taken.

INFANTS AND CHILDREN

A normal temperature taken rectally in infants and small children
is usually below 100°F. Rectal temperatures run about 1° higher than
oral temperatures. (With oral temperatures, cool air entering the
mouth lowers the temperature reading somewhat. The body's temperature, however, is the same throughout the body.)

Children can run high fevers without being seriously ill. It is
always best, however, to report any fever over 101°F to the doctor,
particularly if the child does not feel, look, or act well. Report to the
doctor any other symptoms the child might have.

What to Do
1. It is always best to check with the doctor before giving medication to an infant or small child, particularly one under 1 year of age.
2. Give the child plenty of fluids.
3. Have the child rest, in bed if possible.
4. High fevers (104°F or over) can be reduced by sponging the child with tepid (warm) water and letting the water evaporate on the skin. Recheck the temperature every 25 to 30 minutes. Continue sponge baths until rectal temperature is below 102°F. Be careful, however, that the child does not become chilled.

How to Read a Thermometer
Most temperatures are taken by mouth with an oral (Fahrenheit or Celsius) thermometer. People with mouth injuries, infants, and small children should have their temperature taken by rectum with a rectal thermometer. In oral thermometers, the bulb containing mercury is long and thin; the bulb in a rectal thermometer is short and fat.

To read either type of thermometer, hold the end without the bulb between the thumb and the first finger. Use good light. Look through the pointed edge toward the flat side until you see a thin silver or red line coming out of the bulb. Rotate the

Fahrenheit Thermometer

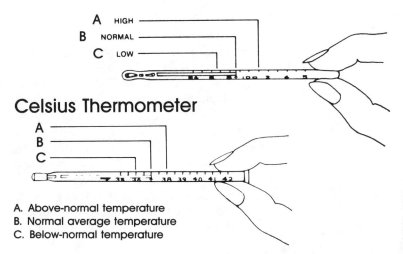

Celsius Thermometer

A. Above-normal temperature
B. Normal average temperature
C. Below-normal temperature

thermometer slightly if the silver line is not visible. The temperature reading is at the end of the silver line. The long lines mark the degrees of temperature and the short lines indicate two-tenths of a degree. An arrow points to the normal reading of 98.6°F (37°C). Readings higher than this indicate a fever, except in a rectal temperature, which is 1° higher.

Before taking a temperature, the thermometer must be shaken down so that the silver or red line reads below the 98.6°F (37°C) mark to approximately 95°F. Hold the thermometer as described above. Shake the thermometer sharply downward with a snapping wrist movement. Read the thermometer to make sure the mercury is shaken down.

How to
Take a
Temperature

If using an oral thermometer, insert the bulb under the victim's tongue. Keep the thermometer in place for at least 3 minutes. Warn the victim not to talk or bite on the thermometer. *Do not* take a temperature for at least 30 minutes after the victim has taken a bath, smoked, eaten hot or cold foods, or drunk water; this can affect the temperature reading.

INJURIES AND ILLNESSES

If you have difficulty reading the thermometer, put it away until someone else can read it. The temperature reading will remain marked until the thermometer is shaken down.

To take a rectal temperature, place the infant or young child on his or her stomach on a firm surface. Separate the buttocks so that the rectum is visible. Lubricate the bulb end of the thermometer with cold cream or petroleum jelly and gently insert into the rectum about 1 inch. Never use force. If you meet resistance, simply change the direction of the thermometer slightly. Put a hand on the child's buttocks and hold the thermometer firmly between your fingers. Leave the thermometer in for 3 minutes. If the child struggles, quiet him or her and place the other hand on the small of his or her back.

FINGERTIP INJURIES (HAMMER-HIT OR DOOR-CRUSH INJURY)

Injuries to the fingertip resulting from a hammer hit or slammed door are extremely painful. Small blood vessels under the fingernail may break, causing a blood clot to form. Within 1 to 2 days, the nail turns black and becomes very painful from the pressure of the blood clot.

NOTE: *It is recommended that a doctor remove the blood clot. However, if medical assistance is not available for a few days and the pain is severe, you can do this yourself by following these instructions.*

What to Do
1. If the blood clot is deep beneath the fingernail, seek medical attention for draining.
2. If the blood clot is close to the tip of the fingernail, it may be drained.
3. Sterilize a needle or paper clip (straightened out) in boiling water for about five minutes or hold over an open flame until red hot.
4. Gently puncture the blood clot to allow draining by inserting the needle point under the fingernail into the clot area. You may have to do this several times in order to break the blood clot.
5. Cover with a sterile bandage.
6. The fingernail should not be pulled off if it becomes loose. Keep the nail in place with a bandage to allow the new fingernail to push off the old one.
7. If the injury is severe, medical attention is recommended for a possible broken bone.

FISHHOOK INJURY

A fishhook caught in the body is a common injury. If the fishhook goes deep enough so that the barb is embedded in the skin, it is best to have a doctor remove it. If a doctor is not readily available, the hook should be removed.

WARNING: *Never* attempt to remove a fishhook caught in the eye or face. Seek medical help immediately.

What to Do

1. If only the point of the hook, and not the barb, entered the skin, remove the hook by backing it out.
2. If the hook is embedded in the skin, push the hook through the skin until the barb comes out.
3. Cut the hook with pliers or clippers at either the barb or the shank of the hook. Remove the part remaining.
4. Clean the wound with soap and water and cover with a bandage.
5. Seek medical attention as soon as possible. In such injuries there is always the possibility of infection, particularly tetanus.

To Remove a Fishhook

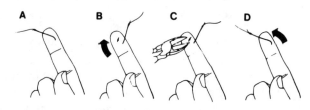

A. The fishhook is embedded beyond the barb in the tip of the finger.
B. Push the hook through the skin until the barb comes out.
C. Cut the hook with pliers or clippers at the barb or at the shank.
D. Carefully remove the remaining part of the hook.

FOOD POISONING

Suspect food poisoning if several people become ill with similar symptoms at approximately the same time after eating the same food. Also suspect food poisoning if one person becomes ill after eating food no one else ate.

BOTULISM

Botulism most often occurs after eating improperly home-canned foods.

WARNING: Botulism is a *very* serious form of food poisoning and is often fatal. It is a medical emergency.

Symptoms   Any or all of the following may be present:

1. Dizziness.
2. Headache.
3. Blurred and/or double vision.
4. Muscle weakness.
5. Difficulty in swallowing.
6. Difficulty in talking.
7. Difficulty in breathing.

Symptoms usually appear within 12 to 36 hours.

Immediate   Seek medical attention immediately, preferably at
Treatment   the nearest hospital emergency room.

MUSHROOM POISONING

Mushroom poisoning occurs after eating certain mushrooms found growing wild.

Symptoms   Any or all of the following may be present:

1. Abdominal pain.   5. Sweating.
2. Diarrhea (may contain blood). 6. Salivation.
3. Vomiting (may contain blood). 7. Tears.
4. Difficulty in breathing.   8. Dizziness.

Symptoms appear within minutes to 24 hours, depending on the type and amount of mushrooms eaten. Symptoms may vary according to the type of mushrooms.

Immediate   1. Call the Poison Control Center, hospital emer-
Treatment   gency room, or doctor for instructions.
              2. Keep the victim resting in a quiet place.
              3. If medical advice is not readily available, in-
                 duce vomiting if vomiting has not already oc-
                 curred. Vomiting may be induced by giving an
                 adult (over 12 years of age unless of low
                 weight) 2 tablespoons of syrup of ipecac; a
                 child between the ages of 1 and 11, 1 table-
                 spoon of syrup of ipecac; an infant under 1
                 year of age, 2 teaspoons. Follow with 1 to 2
                 glasses of water or milk. If vomiting does not
                 occur within 15 to 20 minutes, repeat the do-
                 sage of ipecac *only* once.
              4. *Do not* give mustard or table salt to the victim
                 to induce vomiting.
              5. If syrup of ipecac is not available, induce vom-
                 iting by tickling the back of the victim's throat
                 with your finger or a spoon.
              6. If vomiting does not occur, seek medical atten-
                 tion immediately.
              7. If vomiting occurs, keep the victim face down,
                 head lower than the rest of the body so that he
                 or she will not choke on the vomit. Place a
                 small child face down across your knees.
              8. Seek medical attention immediately.

SALMONELLA POISONING

Salmonella poisoning usually occurs after eating fresh food that has been contaminated with salmonella bacteria. Foods most commonly affected include eggs, milk, raw meats, raw poultry, and raw fish.

Salmonella poisoning can be very serious in infants, young children, the elderly, and the chronically ill.

Symptoms   Any or all of the following may be present:

1. Abdominal cramps.
2. Diarrhea.
3. Fever.
4. Chills.
5. Headache.
6. Vomiting.
7. Weakness.

Symptoms usually appear from 6 to 24 hours after eating contaminated food.

What to Do
1. Keep the victim lying down.
2. Keep the victim comfortably warm.
3. After vomiting is over, give the victim warm mild fluids, such as tea, broth, or fruit juices.
4. Seek medical attention promptly.

STAPHYLOCOCCUS POISONING

Staphylococcus poisoning occurs most often by eating foods that have not been properly refrigerated. The most common foods affected include meats, poultry, eggs, milk, cream-filled bakery goods, tuna and potato salad.

Symptoms   Any or all of the following may be present:

1. Abdominal cramps.
2. Nausea.
3. Vomiting.
4. Diarrhea.

Symptoms usually appear 2 to 6 hours after contaminated food has been eaten.

What to Do
1. Keep the victim resting, preferably in bed.
2. *After* vomiting is over, give the victim warm mild fluids—tea, broth, or fruit juices.
3. It is best to seek medical attention, particularly if the symptoms are severe or persist.

See Also: Abdominal Pain, p. 53; Diarrhea, p. 144; Unconsciousness, p. 251; Vomiting, p. 255.

INJURIES AND ILLNESSES

GAS LEAKS AND OTHER POISONOUS FUMES

Be extremely cautious when rescuing a victim from an area filled with smoke or chemical or gas fumes. It is best not to attempt a rescue alone. Before entering the area, rapidly inhale and exhale two or three times; take a deep breath and hold it. Remain close to the ground (crawl) while entering and rescuing the victim so that you will not inhale hot air or fumes. If the area is extremely hot or heavy with fumes, it is best for the rescuer to have an independent air supply. Do nothing at the site but remove the victim.

ABCs

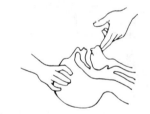

With all serious injuries, check and maintain an open *airway*. Restore *breathing* (p. 20) and *circulation* (p. 22), if necessary.

Immediate Treatment

1. Get the victim into fresh air immediately (upwind of the poisonous fumes).
2. Maintain an open airway. Restore breathing and circulation, if necessary.
3. Loosen tight clothing around the victim's neck and waist.
4. Seek medical attention immediately even if the victim seems to recover completely or partially. Call paramedics, an ambulance, or other trained rescue personnel, and inform medics of the need for oxygen.

HEADACHES

Headaches are a very common complaint. Most headaches are caused by emotional tension and can usually be relieved by aspirin or other similar medication and rest. Applying heat to the back of the neck is often helpful. Massaging the neck muscles and the scalp also helps relieve headache pain.

Other causes of headache include viral infections, sinus infections, allergies, high blood pressure, stroke, brain tumor, meningitis, and head injuries. Any severe or persistent headache requires medical attention.

HEADACHES IN PREGNANCY

Severe or persistent headaches in pregnancy can be a sign of danger to both the mother and the baby. They may indicate a condition known as toxemia, a serious condition in which the mother's body reacts negatively to the presence of the baby. Other symptoms such as swelling in the face and fingers, blurred vision, and rapid weight gain are also usually present. Toxemia occurs during the latter part of the pregnancy. Any severe or persistent headache during pregnancy requires prompt medical attention.

See Also: Drug Abuse, p. 154; Head and Neck Injuries, p. 188; Overexposure: Heat and Cold, p. 209; Poisoning, p. 216; Stroke, p. 246.

INJURIES AND ILLNESSES

HEAD AND NECK INJURIES

For information on neck injury, see p. 191.
For information on cuts of the scalp, see p. 195.

ABCs

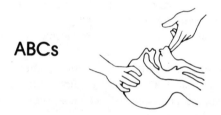

With all serious injuries, check and maintain an open airway. Restore breathing (p. 20) and circulation (p. 22), if necessary.

HEAD INJURIES

WARNING: All head injuries must be taken seriously, as they can result in brain or spinal cord damage. Any victim who is found unconscious must be assumed to have a head injury until determined otherwise by medical personnel. Most head injuries are caused by a fall, a blow to the head, a collision, or sudden stopping, as in an automobile accident.

Anyone with a head injury may also have a neck injury.

Symptoms   Any or all of the following may be present:

1. A cut, bruise, lump, or depression in the scalp.
2. Possible unconsciousness, confusion, or drowsiness.
3. Bleeding from the nose, ear, or mouth.
4. Clear or bloody fluid flowing from the nose or ears.
5. Pale *or* reddish face.
6. Headache.   (*continued on p. 190*)

Mouth-to-Mouth Resuscitation

If the victim is not breathing and no neck injury is suspected, perform all of the following 4 steps.

If a neck injury is suspected (as in a diving or motorcycle accident, or from a fall from a height) *do not* twist or rotate the head. *Slightly* elevate the chin only to open the airway. Check for foreign material in the mouth. Then continue with steps 3 and 4, below.*

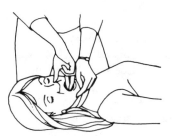

1. Make sure the victim is on a hard, flat surface. Quickly clear the mouth and airway of foreign material.

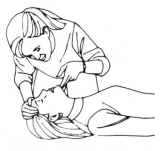

2. Tilt the victim's head backward by placing the palm of your hand on his or her forehead and the fingers of your other hand under the bony part of the chin.

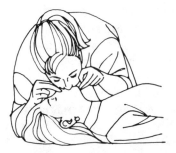

3. Pinch the victim's nostrils with your thumb and index finger. Take a deep breath. Place your mouth tightly over the victim's mouth (mouth and nose for an infant or small child). Give 2 quick breaths.

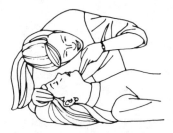

4. Stop blowing when the chest is expanding. Remove your mouth from the victim's mouth and turn your head toward the victim's chest, so that your ear is over his or her mouth. *Listen* for air being exhaled. *Watch* for the victim's chest to fall. Repeat the breathing procedure.

*To move a victim with a neck injury, see p. 191.

INJURIES AND ILLNESSES

(*continued from p. 188*)

7. Vomiting.
8. Convulsions.
9. Pupils of the eyes unequal in size.
10. Difficulty in speech.
11. Restlessness and (possibly) confused behavior.
12. Change in the pulse rate.

Some symptoms may not occur immediately.

Immediate Treatment

1. Maintain an open airway. Be very careful, as there may be a possibility of a broken neck. Restore breathing if necessary by mouth-to-mouth resuscitation.
2. Keep the victim lying down and quiet. If you must move the victim, handle him or her very carefully.
3. If there is no evidence of a neck or back injury, turn the victim's head to the side to allow secretions to drain.
4. Control serious bleeding. (See Bleeding, pp. 80–86.) Gently apply a compress to the bleeding area and bandage it in place.
5. *Do not* give the victim anything by mouth.
6. Seek medical attention promptly, preferably at the nearest hospital emergency room. If someone other than trained medical personnel must take the victim to the hospital, transport the victim lying down, *face up.* Place pads or other suitable material on each side of the victim's head to keep it from moving side to side.

Continued Care

1. Keep the victim comfortably warm.
2. Keep notes on the length and extent of unusual behavior or unconsciousness.

NOTE: *All victims of head injuries should seek prompt medical attention, particularly if the victim was or is unconscious. However, if the victim did not lose consciousness at the time of the injury and did not seek medical attention, delayed symptoms of brain damage* *should be watched for closely for several days. If any of the symptoms of brain damage appear, particularly unconsciousness, change in pulse, difficulty in breathing, convulsions, severe vomiting, eye pupils of unequal size, or a generally poor or ill appearance, medical attention must be sought promptly.*

NECK INJURY

A neck injury should be suspected if a head injury has occurred. *Never* move a victim with a suspected neck injury without trained medical assistance unless the victim is in imminent danger of death (from fire, explosion, or a collapsing building, for example).

WARNING: *Any* movement of the head, either forward, backward, or side to side, can result in paralysis or death.

Symptoms   Any or all of the following may be present:

1. Head injury.
2. Headache.
3. Stiff neck.
4. Inability to move.
5. Inability to move specific parts of the body, such as arms or legs.
6. Tingling sensation in feet and hands.

If the Victim Must Be Moved Because of Immediate Danger to His or Her Life:

Immediate   1.   Immobilize the neck with a rolled towel or
Treatment   newspaper about 4 inches wide wrapped
                   around the neck and tied loosely in place. (*Do not* allow the tie to interfere with victim's breathing.) If the victim is being rescued from an automobile or from water, place a reasonably short, wide board behind the victim's head and back. The board should extend to the victim's buttocks. If possible, tie the board to the victim's body around the forehead and under the armpits. Move the victim very slowly and gently. *Do not* let the victim's body bend or twist.

2. If the victim is not breathing or is having great difficulty in breathing, tilt his or her head *slightly* backward to provide and maintain an open airway.
3. Restore breathing (p. 20) and circulation (p. 22), if necessary.
4. Summon paramedics or trained ambulance personnel immediately.
5. Lay folded towels, blankets, clothing, sandbags, or other suitable objects around the victim's head, neck, and shoulders to keep the head and neck from moving. Place bricks or stones next to the blankets for additional support.
6. Keep the victim comfortably warm.

If the Victim Must Be Taken to the Hospital by Someone Other Than Trained Medical Personnel:

What to Do

1. The victim must be transported lying down on his or her back *face up,* unless there is danger of vomiting, in which case the victim's entire body must be rolled together on its side, keeping the head in the same relationship to the body as it was found.
2. Place a well-padded, rigid support such as a door, table leaf, or wide board next to the victim. Slide the ties under the support.
3. If the victim is breathing on his or her own, hold the victim's head so that it stays in the same relationship to the body as it was found. Other helpers should grasp the victim's clothes and *slide* the victim onto the support. Move the entire body together as a unit.
4. Place folded towels, blankets, or cloths around the victim's head and neck to keep them from moving.
5. If possible, tie the victim's body to the support.
6. Drive carefully to prevent further injury.

Immobilizing a Broken Neck

Never move a victim with a suspected neck injury without trained medical assistance unless the victim is in imminent danger of death (from fire, an explosion, or a collapsing building, for example).

Any movement of the head, either forward, backward, or from side to side, can result in paralysis or death.

Immobilizing a Broken Neck

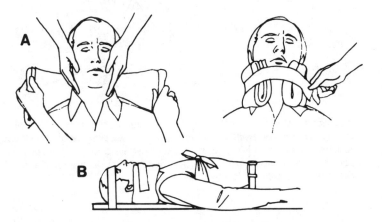

A. Carefully wrap a towel, sweater, newspaper, or some other cushioned item, about 4 inches wide, around the victim's neck, keeping the head as still as possible.

B. Tie the wrap in place, being careful not to interfere with the victim's breathing. If the victim is being rescued from an automobile or from water, place a board behind the victim's head and back. The board should extend to the victim's buttocks. If possible, tie the board to the victim's body around the forehead and under the armpits. Move the victim slowly.

To Move a Victim with a Head or Neck Injury

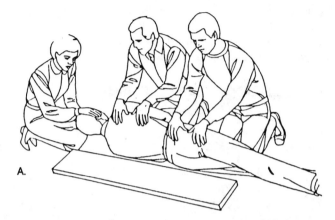

A.

A. If the victim with suspected head or neck injury must be taken to the hospital by someone other than trained medical personnel, the victim must be transported lying down. Place a well-padded rigid support, such as a door or table leaf, next to the victim. The support should extend from beyond the head to the buttocks.

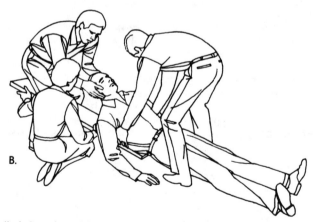

B.

B. The victim's head must be held so that it stays in the same relationship to the body as it was found. Helpers should grasp the victim's clothes and *slide* victim onto the support. Move the entire body as a unit.

SCALP CUTS

Cuts of the scalp may bleed heavily even if the wound is minor.

If the Cut Is **Severe** *or There Is the Possibility of a* **Skull Fracture:**

Immediate
Treatment

1. *Do not* clean the wound or remove any foreign bodies from the scalp.
2. Gently apply a sterile compress and bandage it in place. If bleeding persists, apply pressure firmly about the wound until the bleeding stops.
3. Seek medical attention promptly.

If the Cut Is **Minor:**

What to Do

1. Control the bleeding with pressure.
2. Clean the wound with soap and water.
3. Apply a bandage.

NOTE: *With any cut or puncture, the victim should consult a physician about the necessity for a tetanus shot.*

See Also: Broken Bones and Spinal Injuries, p. 93; Convulsions, p. 133; Dental Emergencies, p. 140; Ear Injuries and Earaches, p. 162; Eye Injuries, p. 169; Unconsciousness, p. 251; Wounds, p. 257.

INJURIES AND ILLNESSES

HEART ATTACK

A heart attack is a life-threatening emergency. It occurs when there is not enough blood and oxygen reaching a portion of the heart due to a narrowing or obstruction of the coronary arteries that supply the heart muscle. If this lack of blood and oxygen is prolonged, a part of the heart muscle will die.

Symptoms   Any or all of the following may be present:

1. Central chest pain that is severe, crushing (not sharp), constant, and lasts for several minutes. Pain may be mistaken for indigestion.
2. Chest discomfort that moves through the chest to either arm, shoulder, neck, jaw, mid-back, or pit of stomach.
3. Profuse sweating.
4. Nausea and vomiting.
5. Extreme weakness.
6. Victim is anxious and afraid.
7. Skin is pale. Fingernails and lips may be blue.
8. Extreme shortness of breath.

If the Victim Is **Unconscious** *and* **Not Breathing,** *or Is Having Difficulty in Breathing:*

(If victim is conscious, see p. 198.)

Immediate   1. Maintain an open airway. Restore breathing
Treatment   and circulation, if necessary.

(*continued on p. 198*)

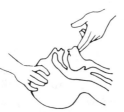

ABCs

With all serious injuries, check and maintain an open *a*irway. Restore *b*reathing (p. 20) and *c*irculation (p. 22), if necessary.

Mouth-to-Mouth Resuscitation

If the Victim Is Not Breathing:

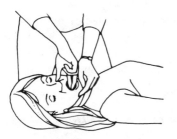

1. Make sure the victim is on a hard, flat surface. Quickly clear the mouth and airway of foreign material.

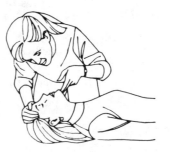

2. Tilt the victim's head backward by placing the palm of your hand on his or her forehead and the fingers of your other hand under the bony part of the chin.

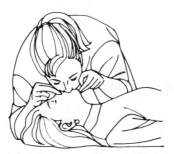

3. Pinch the victim's nostrils with your thumb and index finger. Take a deep breath. Place your mouth tightly over the victim's mouth (mouth and nose for an infant or small child). Give 2 quick breaths.

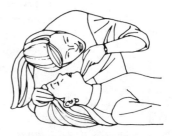

4. Stop blowing when the chest is expanding. Remove your mouth from the victim's mouth and turn your head toward the victim's chest, so that your ear is over his or her mouth. *Listen* for air being exhaled. *Watch* for the victim's chest to fall. Repeat the breathing procedure.

(*continued from p. 196*)

If the Victim Is Conscious at the Onset of the Heart Attack:

Immediate
Treatment

1. Gently place the victim in a comfortable position. This will either be sitting up or in a semi-sitting position. A pillow or two may provide greater comfort. The victim should not lie down flat, as this position makes breathing more difficult.
2. Loosen tight clothing, particularly around the victim's neck.
3. Keep the victim comfortably warm by covering his or her body with a blanket or coat.
4. Calm and reassure the victim.
5. Call an ambulance or paramedics and inform medics of a possible heart attack and of the need for oxygen. If this is not possible, take the victim to the nearest hospital emergency room or physician promptly.

If You Are Alone and Think You're Having a Heart Attack:

What to Do

1. Call an ambulance or paramedics immediately and inform the medics of a possible heart attack and of the need for oxygen.
2. Get into a comfortable position. This will be either sitting up or in a semisitting position. A pillow or two may provide greater comfort.
3. Loosen tight clothing, particularly around your neck.
4. Keep yourself comfortably warm.
5. Do not eat or drink anything.

NOTE: *Not all chest pains are symptoms of a heart attack. Chest pains can be due to strenuous exercise, inflamed nerves, infections, muscle spasms, or excitement. These pains are usually sharp and may repeat but usually last only a few seconds. Chest pains may also be caused by tension, pneumonia, fractured ribs, gas, bruises, strained muscles, or shingles. But it is always a good idea to report any chest pains to a doctor.*

See Also: Shock, p. 234; Unconsciousness, p. 251.

HYPERVENTILATION

Hyperventilation is breathing faster and more deeply than normal due to tension or emotional upset. The victim feels as if he or she is not getting enough air into the lungs and may complain of tightness in the throat. Feeling out of breath, the victim increases respirations in an attempt to take in more air. As rapid breathing continues, the level of carbon dioxide in the blood is lowered, causing muscle tightness in the throat and chest, which further aggravates the symptoms.

Symptoms   Any or all of the following may be present:

1. Lightheadedness.
2. Numbness and tingling in the hands and feet and around the mouth and lips.
3. Possible muscle twitching.
4. Possible difficulty in getting a deep, "satisfying" breath.
5. Possible convulsions.

What to Do
1. If certain of the condition, place a paper bag loosely over the victim's nose and mouth so he or she can rebreathe the air and carbon dioxide mixture, causing the muscles to relax. Have the victim breathe in and out of the bag for four to five minutes. Breathing out (exhaling) should be done slowly.
2. Seek medical attention if breathing does not return to normal. It is also a good idea to suggest seeing a doctor to determine the underlying cause of hyperventilation.

See Also: Convulsions, p. 133.

LEAD POISONING

Lead poisoning most often occurs in young children who nibble on paint chips, plaster, putty, and other substances containing lead.

Symptoms
1. Vomiting.
2. Weakness.
3. Fatigue.
4. Irritability.
5. Fever.
6. Paleness.
7. Convulsions.

WARNING: Brain damage may result from prolonged exposure to lead poisoning.

It is *extremely* important to seek medical attention as soon as lead poisoning is suspected.

See Also: Abdominal Pain, p. 53; Convulsions, p. 133; Rashes, p. 226; Unconsciousness, p. 251; Vomiting, p. 255.

LIGHTNING STRIKE

Being struck by lightning is a serious accident in which the victim's heart can stop beating. The electricity generated by lightning disrupts the electrical activity in the brain that controls breathing and heartbeat. Heat generated by the lightning can also cause severe burns and internal injuries, and broken bones can occur from sudden, strenuous muscle contractions. The victim may also be thrown into the air from the force of the lightning strike.

You can touch a person who has been struck by lightning because the source of the electrical power has dissipated.

Symptoms   Any or all of the following may be present:

1. Disorientation, dizziness.
2. Inability to speak.
3. Unconsciousness.
4. Victim may have stopped breathing.
5. Burn marks.
6. Bleeding.
7. Shock.
8. If the victim was thrown by the force of the lightning, he or she may have suffered additional injuries.

ABCs

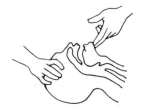

With all serious injuries, check and maintain an open airway. Restore breathing (p. 20) and circulation (p. 22), if necessary.

Immediate Treatment

1. Maintain an open airway. Restore breathing (p. 20) and circulation (p. 22), if necessary.
2. Treat for bleeding, p. 80.
3. Treat for shock, p. 234.
4. Treat any broken bones, p. 93.
5. Calm and reassure the victim.
6. Seek medical attention promptly.

LUMPS AND BUMPS

Lumps and bumps are common injuries. Any bump on the head resulting from an injury may be serious and requires medical attention.

Immediate Treatment

1. As soon as the injury occurs, apply cold compresses or an ice pack to the affected area to decrease swelling and alleviate pain.
2. Seek medical attention promptly for a lump on the head if there is bleeding from the ears, nose, or mouth, unconsciousness, a change in pulse, severe headache, difficulty in breathing, convulsions, severe vomiting, eye pupils of unequal size, slurred speech, a generally poor appearance, or a personality change.
3. If a bump is a result of a head injury, check or awaken the victim every ½ hour for the first 2 hours, every 2 hours for the next 24 hours, every 4 hours for the second 24-hour period, and every 8 hours for the third 24-hour period. By doing this, you are checking to be sure that the victim has not become unconscious.
4. Seek medical attention for any severe lump or bump on any part of the body.

See Also: Broken Bones and Spinal Injuries, p. 93; Bruises, p. 108; Eye Injuries (Blunt Injuries), p. 170; Headaches, p. 187; Head and Neck Injuries, p. 188; Unconsciousness, p. 251.

LYME DISEASE

Lyme disease, named for its discovery in Old Lyme, Connecticut, is a bacterial infection transmitted by the bite of a tick *(Ixodes dammini)*. The tick thrives in wooded and grassy areas throughout the United States and feeds most often on deer and the white-footed mouse. It then transmits the bacterium that causes the disease to humans. The worst months for tick infestation are May through August.

Recent medical studies suggest that the tick must bite for several hours to transmit the disease. (You may not feel the tick biting you.)

Children and adults who live near wooded and grassy areas or who camp or hike near them are most susceptible. Family pets can transport ticks into the home.

Lyme disease is *not* life-threatening, but it can be debilitating. The disease can be successfully treated with antibiotics.

NOTE: *Although* very *uncommon, cases have been reported in which Lyme disease has been passed from a pregnant woman to the fetus.*

Symptoms   Any or all of the following may be present:

1. A round, red rash at the site of the bite. (Children and some adults *may not* develop the rash.)
2. Fever.
3. Chills.
4. Headache.
5. Stiff neck.
6. Fatigue.
7. Muscle and joint pain.
8. Dizziness.

Some symptoms may not appear for several days or months after the victim has been bitten.

Immediate Treatment	1. If you have been bitten by a tick or *suspect* that you have been bitten, see your physician to determine proper treatment. 2. You will most likely be given a blood test. If the test proves negative, as it may in the early stages of the disease, you may be advised to return for additional blood tests. 3. The disease can be successfully treated with antibiotics.

In untreated cases, the disease can, over time, cause heart irregularities, muscle weakness or numbness in the face and limbs, sensitivity to touch, arthritis, and meningitis (inflammation of the membranes that cover the brain and spinal cord). Meningitis causes severe headaches, lethargy, and a stiff neck.

If any of these symptoms develop, seek medical attention promptly.

The tick itself is small, about ⅛ inch in length. (The young tick in its nymphal stage is very small, about the size of a pinhead.) The tick attaches itself to the skin with its mouth and becomes engorged with blood, expanding to 5 to 7 times its original size.

To Remove a Tick from the Skin:

What to Do	1. Using tweezers, gently but firmly grasp the tick at its head and pull it off slowly. 2. *Do not* attempt to pull off the tick with your fingers. The head may break off from the body and embed itself in the skin. 3. *Do not* use a match or lighted cigarette. The heat may cause the tick to embed itself even farther. 4. Clean the wound with an antiseptic or with rubbing alcohol.

If the tick head becomes embedded in the skin:

What to Do	1. Lift up the outer layer of skin with the embedded tick head.

INJURIES AND ILLNESSES

2. Using a sharp, sterilized razor blade, carefully trim or scrape off the skin containing the head *and mouth.* Or use a sterilized needle to break the skin and remove the head and mouth.
3. Clean the wound with an antiseptic or with rubbing alcohol.
4. If you do not want to remove the tick head yourself, see your physician.

Lyme Disease Tick

The tick is small, about ⅛ inch in length. (The young tick in its nymphal stage is very small, about the size of a pinhead.) The tick attaches itself to the skin with its mouth and, engorged with blood, expands to 5 to 7 times its original size.

The Best Treatment for Lyme Disease Is Prevention:

1. Always wear shoes and socks while camping or hiking.
2. Wear long pants and socks *over* the bottom of your pants.
3. Wear a long-sleeved shirt.
4. Wear light-colored clothing so that ticks can be seen.
5. Check regularly for ticks and brush yourself and companions with a broom or towel after hiking.
6. Comb or brush your hair after hiking.
7. Keep towels and clothing off the ground at camping areas and at the beach.
8. Walk on marked trails.
9. Use an insect repellent with chemicals formulated to ward off ticks.
10. Check with your veterinarian for sprays or powders to use on pets.

MISCARRIAGE

A miscarriage is the loss of a fetus before the twentieth week of pregnancy. Miscarriages are common and occur in approximately 10 percent of pregnancies.

The first signs of a possible miscarriage are usually bleeding followed by lower abdominal cramping. Although vaginal bleeding and/or cramping do not always result in a miscarriage, if either of these symptoms appears your doctor should be notified immediately. If heavy or continuous bleeding occurs, seek medical attention immediately, preferably at the nearest hospital emergency room.

Until the doctor is notified and can give specific instructions, the woman should rest in bed. If any material resembling the fetus (tissue or unusual-looking clots) is passed from the vagina, it should be saved (preferably in a container in the refrigerator) for inspection by the doctor.

See Also: Abdominal Pain, p. 53; Childbirth, Emergency, p. 119; Pregnancy, Danger Signs, p. 221.

INJURIES AND ILLNESSES

MUSCLE ACHES AND PAINS

Pain in the muscles is common and usually not serious. These pains are often caused by tension, infections, fatigue (particularly in children), and overexercising. Gently massaging the area, applying heat by means of a warm bath or warm wet compresses, and resting are often helpful in relieving the pain. Stretching exercises begun slowly also may be helpful. Any pain that is severe or prolonged needs medical attention.

Muscle cramps can be particularly painful and often occur in the middle of the night. They usually result from fatigue or from keeping the limb in one position for a prolonged period. Muscle cramps often occur in the foot, the calf of the leg, and the thigh. Massaging the area to relax the muscle is usually effective, because it stimulates local circulation.

If the cramp is in the foot, turn the toes up toward your body and bend the foot back. If the cramp is in the calf of the leg, stand up with most of your weight on the unaffected leg and massage the cramp. For a cramp in the thigh, lie down while massaging the area. Heat is often helpful.

Cramps in the legs and thighs often occur during pregnancy. The treatment is the same as described for muscle cramps. Also, be sure to get plenty of rest.

See Also: Bites and Stings (Multiple Stings, Black Widow Spider Bites), pp. 67, 68; Broken Bones and Spinal Injuries, p. 93; Bruises, p. 108; Dislocations, p. 147; Food Poisoning, p. 183; Overexposure: Heat and Cold (Heat Cramps, Heat Exhaustion), pp. 209, 210; Sprains, p. 243; Strains, p. 245; and Part III: Sports First Aid, p. 267–319.

OVEREXPOSURE: HEAT AND COLD

HEAT INJURIES

Heat Cramps

Heat cramps are muscle pains and spasms caused by a loss of salt from the body due to profuse sweating. Strenuous physical activity in hot temperatures can lead to heat cramps. Usually the muscles of the stomach and legs are affected first. Heat cramps may also be a symptom of heat exhaustion.

ABCs

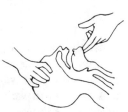

With all serious injuries, check and maintain an open airway. Restore breathing (p. 20) and circulation (p. 22), if necessary.

Symptoms   Any or all of the following may be present:

1. Painful muscle cramping and spasms.
2. Heavy sweating.
3. Possible convulsions.

What to Do   1. Have the victim sit quietly in a cool place.
2. Apply firm hand pressure to the affected area or gently massage the victim's cramped muscles.

3. If the victim is not vomiting, give clear juice or sips of cool salt water (1 teaspoon of salt per glass). Give victim ½ glass of liquid every 15 minutes for 1 hour. Stop fluids if vomiting occurs.
4. Medical attention is needed if available because of other possible complications.

Heat Exhaustion

Heat exhaustion can occur after prolonged exposure to high temperatures and high humidity.

Symptoms   Any or all of the following may be present:

1. Body temperature normal or slightly above normal.
2. Pale and clammy skin.
3. Heavy sweating.
4. Tiredness, weakness.
5. Dizziness.
6. Headache.
7. Nausea.
8. Possible muscle cramps.
9. Possible vomiting.
10. Possible fainting.

What to Do
1. Move the victim into the shade or to a cooler area.
2. Have the victim lie down.
3. Raise the victim's feet 8 to 12 inches.
4. Loosen the victim's clothing.
5. If the victim is not vomiting, give clear juice or sips of cool salt water (1 teaspoon of salt per glass). Give the victim ½ glass of liquid every 15 minutes for 1 hour. Stop fluids if vomiting occurs.
6. Place cool wet cloths on the victim's forehead and body.
7. Use a fan to cool the victim or, if possible, remove the victim to an air-conditioned room.
8. If symptoms are severe, become worse, or last longer than an hour, seek medical attention promptly.

Heatstroke (Sunstroke)

Heatstroke is a life-threatening emergency. It is a disturbance in the body's heat-regulating system caused by extremely high body temperature due to exposure to heat and from an inability of the body to cool itself.

Symptoms   Any or all of the following may be present:

1. Extremely high body temperature (often 106°F or higher).
2. Red, hot, and dry skin. Sweating usually absent.
3. Rapid and strong pulse.
4. Possible unconsciousness or confusion.

If Body Temperature Reaches 105°F:

Immediate
Treatment
1. Undress the victim and put him or her into a tub of cold water (not iced) if possible. Otherwise, spray the victim with a hose, sponge bare skin with cool water or rubbing alcohol, or apply cold packs to the victim's body.
2. Continue treatment until body temperature is lowered to 101° or 102°F.
3. Do not overchill. Check temperature constantly.
4. Dry off the victim once temperature is lowered.
5. Seek medical attention promptly, preferably at the nearest hospital emergency room.

Continued
Care
1. Place the victim in front of a fan or an air conditioner to continue cooling.
2. If body temperature rises again, repeat the cooling process.
3. *Do not* give the victim alcoholic beverages or stimulants such as coffee or tea.

Sunburn

Sunburn is usually a first-degree burn of the skin resulting from overexposure to the sun. Prolonged exposure can lead to a second-degree burn.

Symptoms   Any or all of the following may be present:

1. Redness.
2. Pain.

3. Mild swelling.
4. Blisters and considerable swelling in severe cases.

INJURIES AND ILLNESSES

What to Do
1. Put cold water on the sunburned area.
2. If sunburn is severe, submerge the sunburned area under cold water until pain is relieved. It is also helpful to place cold wet cloths on the burned area. Do not rub the skin.
3. Elevate severely sunburned arms or legs.
4. If possible, put a dry sterile bandage on severely sunburned area.
5. Seek medical attention for severe sunburn. *Do not* break blisters or put ointments, sprays, antiseptic medications, or home remedies on severe sunburns.

COLD INJURIES

Frostbite

Frostbite is the freezing of parts of the body due to exposure to very low temperatures. Frostbite occurs when ice crystals form in the fluid in the cells of the skin and tissues. The toes, fingers, nose, and ears are affected most often.

Symptoms   Any or all of the following may be present:

1. In the earliest stages skin appears red. Pain is often present.
2. As frostbite develops, skin becomes white or grayish yellow and appears and feels waxy and firm.
3. Skin feels very cold and numb.
4. Pain disappears.
5. Blisters may form.
6. Often the victim is not aware of frostbite until someone else notices the above symptoms.

Immediate Treatment
1. While outside, cover the frozen part with extra clothing or a warm cloth. If the hand or fingers are frostbitten, put the hand under the armpit for additional warmth.
2. *Do not* rub the frostbitten part with snow or anything else.
3. Bring the victim inside promptly.
4. The frostbitten area must be rewarmed rapidly. Put the victim's frostbitten part in *warm* (not hot) water that is between 100° and

104°F. Test the water with a thermometer or by applying it to your forearm.

5. If warm water is not available, gently wrap the frostbitten part in blankets or other warm materials.

6. *Do not* use heat lamps, hot water bottles, or heating pads.

7. *Do not* allow the victim to place the frostbitten part near a hot stove or radiator. Frostbitten parts may become burned before feeling returns.

8. *Do not* break blisters.

9. Stop the warming process when the skin becomes pink and/or feeling begins to come back.

10. Seek medical attention promptly.

Continued Care

1. Give the victim warm drinks such as tea, coffee, or soup.

2. *Do not* give alcoholic beverages.

3. Have the victim exercise fingers or toes as soon as they are warmed.

4. *Do not* allow a victim with frostbitten feet or toes to walk. This may cause further damage to the frostbitten part.

5. Put sterile gauze between frostbitten fingers or toes to keep them separated.

6. Keep the frostbitten parts elevated, if possible.

7. Take extreme care that the frostbitten area is not refrozen after it has thawed.

Danger Signals

If severe frostbite has occurred, the victim may not have feeling in the frostbitten areas and they may be black in color, meaning that the skin tissue has died.

WARNING: If severe frostbite has occurred, cover the frostbitten areas with warm materials and take the victim *without delay* to the nearest hospital emergency room for treatment.

INJURIES AND ILLNESSES

Hypothermia (Chilling and Freezing of Entire Body)

Symptoms   Any or all of the following may be present:

1. Shivering.
2. Numbness.
3. Drowsiness, sleepiness.
4. Muscle weakness.
5. Low body temperature.
6. Unconsciousness if entire body is severely chilled or frozen.

Immediate
Treatment

1. Maintain an open airway and restore breath ing if necessary (see p. 20).
2. Bring the victim into a warm room as soon as possible.
3. Remove wet clothes.
4. Wrap the victim in warm blankets, towels, additional clothing, or sheets.
5. Seek medical attention promptly.

Continued
Care

1. If the victim is conscious, give him or her comfortably warm drinks such as coffee, tea, or soup.
2. *Do not* give the victim alcoholic beverages.
3. See treatment and care for frostbite, p. 212.

Mild Chilling

For mild chilling put the victim in a warm room and wrap in warm blankets. Give the victim warm drinks such as coffee, tea, or soup. *Do not* give the victim alcoholic beverages.

See Also: Burns, p. 109; Convulsions, p. 133; Dehydration, p. 139; Drowning, p. 148; Ear Injuries and Earaches (Frostbite), p. 164; Fever, p. 177; Unconsciousness, p. 251.

PLANT IRRITATIONS (POISON IVY, POISON OAK, AND POISON SUMAC)

An oily substance on the plants causes the irritation.

Symptoms   Any or all of the following may be present:

1. Redness of the skin.
2. Blisters.
3. Itching.
4. Headache.
5. Fever.

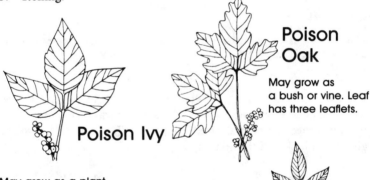

Poison Ivy

Poison Oak

May grow as a bush or vine. Leaf has three leaflets.

May grow as a plant, bush, or vine. Leaf has three shiny leaflets.

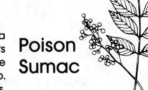

May grow as a bush or tree. Leaf consists of rows of two leaflets opposite each other plus a leaflet at top. Leaflets are pointed at both ends.

Poison Sumac

What to Do
1. As soon as possible, remove clothes and thoroughly wash the affected area with soap and water.
2. Sponge the affected area with rubbing alcohol.
3. Calamine lotion may be applied to relieve itching.

POISONING

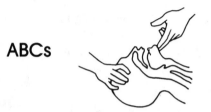

ABCs

With all serious injuries, check and maintain an open *a*irway. Restore *b*reathing (p. 20) and *c*irculation (p. 22), if necessary.

It is extremely important to call a Poison Control Center (if available), a hospital emergency room, a doctor, or paramedics for instructions if someone has swallowed a poison. When calling, be sure to give the following information:

1. The victim's age.
2. Name of the poison.
3. How much poison was swallowed.
4. When poison was swallowed.
5. Whether or not the victim has vomited.
6. How much time it will take to get the victim to a medical facility.

Emergency treatment for victims of swallowed poisons consists of:

1. Diluting the poison with water or milk as quickly as possible. *Do not* give fruit juice or vinegar to neutralize the poison.
2. Getting the poison out of the victim by induced vomiting (on medical advice only—preferably from the staff at a Poison Control Center).
3. Seeking prompt medical attention.

WARNING: *Never* give liquids to dilute the poison or induce vomiting if the victim is unconscious or is having convulsions. Also, *do not induce vomiting* if you do not know what the victim has swallowed.

Do not induce vomiting if the victim has swallowed:

1. A strong ACID or ALKALI such as toilet bowl cleaner, rust removers, chlorine bleach, dishwasher detergent, or glucose-test tablets.
2. A PETROLEUM PRODUCT such as kerosene, gasoline, furniture polish, charcoal lighter fluid, or paint thinner.

Give water, not milk, with any of these products.

Strong acids and alkalis, if vomited, may cause further damage to the throat and esophagus. Petroleum products, if vomited, can be drawn into the lungs and cause a chemical pneumonia. It is important to note, however, that a Poison Control Center may recommend induced vomiting for some of the above-mentioned products (particularly the petroleum products) because of other chemicals in the swallowed product that may be more harmful to the body.

Always follow the instructions of the Poison Control Center.

If the victim vomits, whether induced or spontaneously, keep the victim's face down with the head lower than the rest of the body so that he or she will not choke on the vomit. Place a small child face down across your knees. *Be sure* to take the poison container and any vomited material to the hospital for inspection.

NOTE: *Antidotes on labels of poisonous substances are not always correct, particularly if the container is old. It is always best to consult a Poison Control Center if possible.*

If the Victim Is Not Breathing:

Immediate Treatment	1. Maintain an open airway.
	2. Restore breathing (p. 20) and circulation (p. 22), if necessary.
	3. Seek medical attention immediately. Call paramedics, an ambulance, the fire department, or other rescue personnel for transportation to the hospital.
	4. Take the poison container and any vomited material to the hospital with the victim.

INJURIES AND ILLNESSES

If the Victim Is Unconscious *or* Having Convulsions:

Immediate
Treatment

1. Maintain an open airway if possible. Restore breathing if necessary.
2. Loosen tight clothing around the victim's neck and waist.
3. Seek medical attention immediately. Call paramedics, an ambulance, the fire department, or other rescue personnel for transportation to the hospital. The victim should be transported lying on his or her side or stomach.
4. Take the poison container and any vomited material to the hospital with the victim.
5. *Do not* give any fluids to the victim.
6. *Do not* try to induce vomiting. If the victim vomits on his or her own, turn the victim's head to the side so that he or she will not choke on the vomit.

If the Victim Is Conscious:

Immediate
Treatment

1. Immediately give the victim at least one 8-ounce glass of water or milk (give only water with gasoline products) to dilute the poison. *Do not* give fruit juice, vinegar, carbonated drinks, or alcohol to neutralize the poison.
2. Have someone else (if possible) call the Poison Control Center, hospital emergency room, or doctor for further instructions while you continue to care for the victim.
3. Induce vomiting *only* if told to do so by one of the above-listed medical personnel. If no medical advice is readily available, induce vomiting only if the swallowed poison is *not* an acid, alkali, or petroleum product. Vomiting may be induced by giving an adult (over 12 years of age unless of low weight) 2 tablespoons of syrup of ipecac; a child between the ages of 1 to 11, 1 tablespoon of syrup of ipecac; an infant under 1 year of age, 2 teaspoons. Follow with 1 to 2 glasses of water or milk. If vomiting does

(*continued on p. 220*)

Mouth-to-Mouth Resuscitation

If the Victim Is Not Breathing:

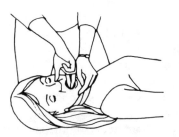

1. Make sure the victim is on a hard, flat surface. Quickly clear the mouth and airway of foreign material.

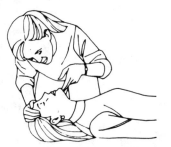

2. Tilt the victim's head backward by placing the palm of your hand on his or her forehead and the fingers of your other hand under the bony part of the chin.

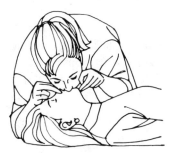

3. Pinch the victim's nostrils with your thumb and index finger. Take a deep breath. Place your mouth tightly over the victim's mouth (mouth and nose for an infant or small child). Give 2 quick breaths.

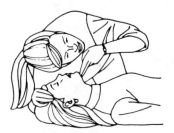

4. Stop blowing when the chest is expanding. Remove your mouth from the victim's mouth and turn your head toward the victim's chest, so that your ear is over his or her mouth. *Listen* for air being exhaled. *Watch* for the victim's chest to fall. Repeat the breathing procedure.

INJURIES AND ILLNESSES

(*continued from p. 218*)
not occur within 15 to 20 minutes, repeat dosage of ipecac *only* once.

4.   *Do not* give mustard or table salt to the victim to induce vomiting.

5.   If syrup of ipecac is not available, induce vomiting by tickling the back of the victim's throat with your finger or a spoon.

6.   If vomiting does not occur, seek medical attention immediately.

7.   If vomiting occurs, keep the victim face down with the head lower than the rest of the body so that he or she will not choke on the vomit. Place a small child face down across your knees.

8.   Seek medical attention immediately. Take the poison container and any vomited material to the hospital with the victim.

See Also: Abdominal Pain, p. 53; Burns (Chemical Burns), p. 114; Convulsions, p. 133; Diarrhea, p. 144; Drug Abuse, p. 154; Food Poisoning, p. 183; Gas Leaks and Other Poisonous Fumes, p. 186; Lead Poisoning, p. 200; Rashes, p. 226; Unconsciousness, p. 251.

PREGNANCY, DANGER SIGNS

Certain symptoms during pregnancy should be reported immediately to a doctor. They may or may not indicate a serious condition, but only a doctor can evaluate the situation. The symptoms to report immediately include:

1. *Any* vaginal bleeding.
2. Stomach pain or cramps.
3. Persistent vomiting.
4. Severe, persistent headaches.
5. Swelling of the face or fingers.
6. Blurring or dimness of vision.
7. Chills and fever.
8. Sudden leaking of water from the vagina.
9. Convulsions.

See Also: Abdominal Pain (Ectopic Pregnancy), p. 55; Childbirth, Emergency, p. 119; Miscarriage, p. 207.

RAPE/SEXUAL ASSAULT

Rape or sexual assault occurs when an individual is forced to partici-
pate in sexual activities against his or her wishes. In adults, rape
usually occurs when one or several adults partially or completely
penetrate a woman's vagina or other body opening through forcible
sexual intercourse or with the use of an inanimate object.

Rape also can be perpetrated against children by other children
or by adults. (See Child Abuse (Misuse)/Other Person Abuse, p.
115.)

Rape is a crime in every state. Some state laws have been ex-
panded to include rape in marriage and between individuals of the
same sex. The motives of the rapist are dominance and control.

If you are alone and you have been raped, or if another person has
been raped, call the police immediately to report the crime. Next,
call a relative, a friend, or a rape hotline (or other community agency
with rape counseling available) to assist you. Then call your doctor
or the hospital emergency room to let them know that a rape has
occurred and that you or another individual will be seeking medical
treatment.

Symptoms   Injuries will vary according to the manner in
           which the victim was attacked.
           Any or all of the following may be present:

1. Severe pain.
2. Bleeding.
3. Noticeable signs of physical abuse: cuts, burns, bruises (from
   being hit, choked, strangled, or kicked).
4. If conscious, the victim may be overcome with fear, anxiety, or
   depression, and may suffer from feelings of degradation and
   embarrassment.

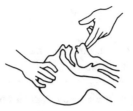

ABCs

With all serious injuries, check for and maintain an open *airway*. Restore *breathing* (p. 20) and *circulation* (p. 22), if necessary.

Immediate Treatment

1. If the victim is unconscious, restore breathing and circulation, if necessary.
2. Stop any severe bleeding. (See Bleeding, p. 80.)
3. Treat any broken bones. (See Broken Bones and Spinal Injuries, p. 93.)
4. Treat for symptoms of shock. (See Shock, p. 234.)
5. Comfort the victim as much as possible.

INJURIES AND ILLNESSES

Do Not Allow the Victim to:

Change clothes. Take a shower. Brush his or her teeth.

Do the Following:

Call the police to report the crime.

Call someone to assist you: a relative, a friend, a rape hotline.

Call your doctor or hospital emergency room.

(*continued on p. 225*)

Mouth-to-Mouth Resuscitation

If the victim is not breathing and no neck injury is suspected, perform all of the following 4 steps.

If a neck injury is suspected (as in a fall from a height) *do not* twist
or rotate the head. *Slightly* elevate the chin only to open the airway.
Check for foreign material in the mouth. Then continue with steps
3 and 4, below.*

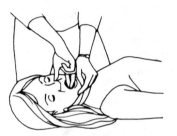

1. Make sure the victim is on a
hard, flat surface. Quickly clear
the mouth and airway of foreign material.

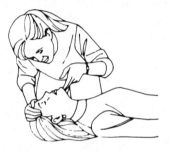

2. Tilt the victim's head backward
by placing the palm of your
hand on his or her forehead
and the fingers of your other
hand under the bony part of
the chin.

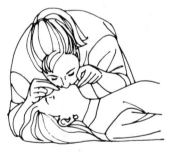

3. Pinch the victim's nostrils with
your thumb and index finger.
Take a deep breath. Place
your mouth tightly over the victim's mouth (mouth and nose
for an infant or small child).
Give 2 quick breaths.

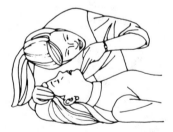

4. Stop blowing when the chest
is expanding. Remove your
mouth from the victim's mouth
and turn your head toward the
victim's chest, so that your ear
is over his or her mouth. *Listen*
for air being exhaled. *Watch*
for the victim's chest to fall. Repeat the breathing procedure.

*To move a victim with a neck injury, see p. 191.

(*continued from p. 223*)
The rape victim will be given a private room or taken to a secluded area at the physician's office or hospital emergency room. A rape counselor, policeman or policewoman, and medical personnel may all be present to help. The victim may be asked several times to describe what happened and to give a description of the assailant.

A physician will recommend that the victim have a complete physical examination. The exam is performed to protect the victim from disease and to establish proof of the claim that the rape occurred.

The exam will include taking cultures (samples) from the mouth, vagina, and rectum, and tests for infections such as chlamydia, gonorrhea, and syphilis. Additional tests may be taken for pregnancy, and, possibly, for AIDS. The tests will determine the victim's health status for these conditions at the time the crime occurred.

Continued Care

1. Have someone stay with the victim. The victim should not stay alone immediately after the rape.
2. If you are taking care of a rape victim, offer your support.
3. Seek follow-up medical treatment, depending upon the injuries, and test results.
4. Seek counseling for assistance in handling the emotional aspects of the rape.

INJURIES AND ILLNESSES

RASHES

Skin rashes occur for many reasons. They may be due to allergic reactions, fever, heat, infectious diseases, or other causes. Some rashes may indicate a serious problem. Medical attention should always be sought if blue, purple, or blood-red spots appear (these may mean bleeding in and under the skin); the rash becomes worse; signs of infection such as pus or red streaks occur; itching is severe; or if other symptoms are present.

BITES AND STINGS

Rashes may appear after insect stings, tick bites, brown recluse spider bites, and rat bites. Rashes that result from bites and stings should be seen by a doctor. Some may rapidly lead to breathing difficulties.

DISEASES

Rashes are present with many infectious diseases. Among these are chicken pox, measles, German (three-day) measles, Rocky Mountain spotted fever, smallpox, scarlet fever, certain forms of meningitis, roseola infantum, and infectious mononucleosis.

DRUG RASH

A skin reaction may appear with any medication, although these rashes are more likely to appear with the use of powerful drugs such as barbiturates, tranquilizers, and antibiotics. If a rash appears while the person is on a medication, call the doctor immediately to see if a rash is to be expected from the illness for which the medication was prescribed, or if it is a reaction to the drug.

HEAT RASH

A common rash is heat rash (also called prickly heat). This rash is caused by high body temperatures due to fever or hot, humid weather. In heat rash the body's sweat ducts are blocked. The area affected is covered with tiny red pinpoints. Treatment consists of avoiding extreme heat.

Dusting powders and soothing lotions are also helpful. Light, dry, and loose clothing should be worn in hot weather. Heat rash usually disappears in a cool environment. If heat rash persists, a doctor should be consulted.

HIVES

Hives are an allergic reaction to various substances characterized by large or small irregularly shaped and sized bumpy swellings that cause stinging, burning, and itching. Animal hairs, feathers, laundry detergents, plants, fabrics, dyes, medications, and viral infections may cause hives. Food is a common offender, particularly chocolate, nuts, berries, and seafood. For first attacks of hives, it is best to seek medical attention. If hives have occurred before, follow previous instructions of the doctor. If hives persist, see your doctor. If other symptoms are present, such as difficulty in breathing or swallowing, seek medical attention promptly.

POISONOUS RASHES

Contact with plants often produces a rash in sensitive persons. The most common offenders are poison ivy, poison oak, and poison sumac. (See Plant Irritations, p. 215.)

RASHES IN INFANTS

Infants often have rashes. The most common is diaper rash. It is not dangerous but can cause a lot of discomfort. Diaper rash usually is

INJURIES AND ILLNESSES

an ammonia burn that occurs when bacteria act upon passed urine that stays on the skin for prolonged periods and break down the urine into ammonia. Diaper rash may also be caused by fungi found in the infant's stools. Thorough skin cleansing followed by drying will help. *Very* absorbent, dry diapers should be used and changed frequently. Various ointments are available, but it is best to ask a doctor for specific instructions.

A common rash in newborns appears during the early weeks of life. It may appear anywhere on the body. It often moves from one place to another. The affected area should be kept clean and dry. It is always a good idea to report all rashes on an infant to a doctor.

Rashes seen on infants are also caused by food allergies and by contact with substances such as clothes washed in strong detergents, rubber in pants, skin care products, and soap left behind the ears. These rashes should also be reported to a doctor.

See Also: Bites and Stings, p. 63; Lyme Disease, p. 204; Rocky Mountain Spotted Fever, p. 229.

ROCKY MOUNTAIN SPOTTED FEVER

Rocky Mountain spotted fever is a serious but rare rickettsial infection transmitted by the bite of a tick *(Dermacentor andersoni)*. The rickettsia is the parasitic microorganism that causes the disease. The tick feeds on small mammals, such as rabbits and rodents, and from them can pass on the rickettsia to humans. Family pets can transport ticks into the home.

Recent medical studies suggest that the tick must bite for several hours to transmit the disease. (You may not feel the tick biting you.)

Although first recognized in the Rocky Mountains, the disease can occur anywhere in the United States and in Canada.

Rocky Mountain spotted fever *can be fatal*. If caught early, however, it can be successfully treated with antibiotics.

Symptoms   Any or all of the following may be present:

1. Headache.
2. Fever (mild to severe).
3. Loss of appetite.
4. Rash—pink to deep red spots—that appears first on the wrists and ankles, then spreads to the palms of the hands, the soles of the feet, the forearms, and then to the rest of the body.
5. Swelling around the eyes and of the inner eyelids.
6. Swelling of the feet and hands.

Some symptoms may not appear for several weeks after the victim has been bitten. In other cases, symptoms may appear suddenly.

Immediate Treatment
1. If you have been bitten by a tick or *suspect* that you have been bitten, see your physician to determine proper treatment.

2. You will most likely be given a blood test. If the test proves negative, you may be asked to return for additional blood tests.
3. The disease can be successfully treated with antibiotics.

The tick attaches itself to the skin with its mouth and becomes engorged with blood.

To Remove a Tick from the Skin:

What to Do
1. Using tweezers, gently but firmly grasp the tick at its head and pull it off slowly.
2. *Do not* attempt to pull off the tick with your fingers. The head may break off from the body and embed itself in the skin.
3. *Do not* use a match or lighted cigarette. The heat may cause the tick to embed itself even farther.
4. Clean the wound with an antiseptic or with rubbing alcohol.

If the Tick Head Becomes Embedded in the Skin:

What to Do
1. Lift up the outer layer of skin with the embedded tick head.
2. Using a sharp, sterilized razor blade, carefully trim or scrape off the skin containing the head *and mouth*. Or use a sterilized needle to break the skin and remove the head and mouth.
3. Clean the wound with an antiseptic or with rubbing alcohol.
4. If you do not want to remove the tick head yourself, see your physician.

The Best Treatment for Rocky Mountain Spotted Fever Is Prevention:

1. Always wear shoes and socks while camping or hiking.
2. Wear long pants and socks *over* the bottom of your pants.
3. Wear a long-sleeved shirt.
4. Wear light-colored clothing so that ticks can be seen.

5. Check regularly for ticks and brush off yourself and companions with a broom or towel after hiking.
6. Comb or brush your hair after hiking.
7. Keep towels and clothing off the ground at camping areas and at the beach.
8. Walk on marked trails.
9. Use an insect repellent with chemicals formulated to ward off ticks.
10. Check with your veterinarian for sprays or powders to use on pets.

INJURIES AND ILLNESSES

SEVERED LIMB

A severed limb is a serious emergency and requires prompt medical attention. A victim who has suffered severing of a limb, such as a finger, hand, arm, or foot, may be bleeding profusely and have other injuries or medical conditions that will need to be treated.

With loss of a limb, the first medical concern is always for the victim. The second concern is for the severed limb, which, in many instances, can be successfully reattached.

Symptoms   Any or all of the following may be present:

1. A large loss of blood.
2. Weakness, dizziness.
3. Vomiting.

4. Shock.
5. Broken bones.
6. Unconsciousness.

ABCs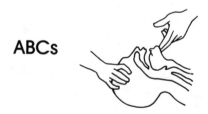

With all serious injuries, check and maintain an open *a*irway. Restore *b*reathing (p. 20) and *c*irculation (p. 22), if necessary.

Immediate Treatment
1. Maintain an open airway. Restore breathing (p. 20) and circulation (p. 22), if necessary.
2. Treat for bleeding. (See Bleeding [External Bleeding—Immediate Treatment], p. 80.)

3. Treat for shock. (See Shock, p. 234.)
4. If the victim is vomiting, turn the victim on his or her side or turn the head sideways, *only if you do not suspect a neck injury,* so that he or she does not choke on the vomit.
5. Seek medical attention promptly, preferably at the nearest hospital emergency room.

To Care for the Severed Limb:

1. *After* you have cared for the victim, place the limb in a clean plastic bag, garbage bag, or other suitable container to keep the limb from drying out and to prevent contamination.
2. Pack ice around the limb on the *outside* of the bag or container to keep the limb cold. The ice must not touch the limb directly and the limb should not soak in ice or water. (If a second bag or container is available, the ice should be placed in this bag. Then place the bag with the limb in it into the bag of ice.) Keeping the limb cold decreases its need for oxygen.
3. Call the hospital to notify them of a victim with a severed limb. Doing so will give the hospital time to prepare for the victim's arrival. If the hospital is not equipped to perform surgical reimplantation, the staff often can make arrangements and will direct the victim to a hospital that is able to perform this procedure.

INJURIES AND ILLNESSES

SHOCK

Shock is a medical condition secondary to serious illness or injury. It is a life-threatening situation in which the body's vital functions, such as breathing and heartbeat, are seriously threatened by insufficient oxygenated blood reaching body tissues, such as the lungs, the brain, and the heart.

SHOCK FROM AN ALLERGIC REACTION TO INSECT STINGS, MEDICATION, OR FOOD (ANAPHYLACTIC SHOCK)

Anaphylactic shock is a life-threatening condition.

Symptoms   Any or all of the following may be present:

1. Weakness.
2. Coughing and/or wheezing.
3. Difficulty in breathing.
4. Severe itching or hives.
5. Severe swelling in other parts of the body and at the bite site.
6. Stomach cramps.
7. Nausea and vomiting.
8. Anxiety.
9. Possible bluish tinge to skin.
10. Dizziness.
11. Collapse.
12. Possible unconsciousness.

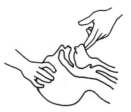

ABCs

With all serious injuries, check and maintain an open *airway*. Restore *b*reathing (p. 20) and *c*irculation (p. 22), if necessary.

Immediate Treatment

1. Maintain an open airway and restore breathing (p. 20) if necessary.
2. If stung by a honeybee, carefully remove the stinger by gently scraping out the stinger with a knife blade, card edge, or fingernail. Removing the stinger reduces the amount of venom entering the body. *Do not* use tweezers or squeeze the stinger while removing it, as this may result in more venom entering the body.

If an Emergency Kit for Insect Stings Is **Not** *Available:*

1. If the victim experiences the severe symptoms above, suggesting a severe allergic reaction, and the victim is known to have had previous severe reactions to insect stings, the use of a tourniquet may be necessary. Although not all experts agree on this method, many allergists recommend the use of a tourniquet in severe reactions where the victim's life is at stake. Emergency insect sting kits available only by prescription contain a tourniquet for such cases. A tourniquet helps to slow the flow of blood and absorption of venom throughout the body.

   The tourniquet is used only if the sting has just occurred and is on the arm or leg. A rubber tourniquet works best but a strip of cloth or cord may be used.

   Tie the tourniquet 2 to 4 inches above the sting, between the sting and the body. *Do not* tie so tightly that the victim's arterial

INJURIES AND ILLNESSES

Light Tourniquet

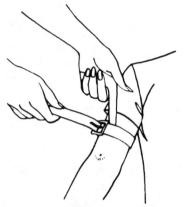

A light constricting band is used for *severe* reactions to insect stings (see Insect Stings, Anaphylactic Shock in text) and for rattlesnake, copperhead, and cottonmouth (not coral) snakebites. A light tourniquet of this sort restricts the blood flow and absorption of venom in the body. Place the band 2 to 4 inches above the bite, between the bite and body. *Do not* cut off arterial circulation. You should be able to slip your finger under the band.

circulation is cut off completely. Loosen the tourniquet about every five minutes until medical assistance is obtained.

2. If the victim experiences severe symptoms of an allergic reaction but has no known previous history of severe reactions to insect stings, and the sting has just occurred on the arm or leg, apply a light constricting band such as an elastic watchband, belt, or tie 2 to 4 inches above the sting, between the sting and the body. The band *should not* be so tight that it cuts off arterial circulation. You should be able to slip your finger under the band. *Do not* remove the band until medical assistance is obtained.

3. Seek medical attention promptly, preferably at the nearest hospital emergency room.

Continued Care

1. Place cold pack or ice wrapped in cloth on sting area. This will help stop absorption and spread of the injected venom.

2. Keep the victim lying down. Turn the victim's head to the side if he or she is vomiting, or position the victim on his or her side.

3. Keep the victim comfortable.

If an Emergency Kit for Insect Stings **Is Available:**

Immediate
Treatment

1. Maintain an open airway and restore breathing (p. 20) if necessary.
2. Remove the stinger if stung by a honeybee. To do this, gently scrape out the stinger with a knife blade, card edge, or fingernail. *Do not* squeeze the stinger with tweezers, as this may result in more venom entering the body.
3. If the victim is unable to administer an injection of adrenaline to himself or herself, follow directions in the emergency kit.
4. Seek medical attention promptly, preferably at the nearest hospital emergency room.

Continued
Care

1. Place cold compresses on the sting area to stop absorption and spread of the injected venom.
2. Keep the victim lying down unless he or she is short of breath; then let the victim sit up slowly.
3. Keep the victim comfortable and quiet.

SHOCK DUE TO INJURY (TRAUMATIC SHOCK)

Traumatic shock occurs with injuries that result in loss of blood, loss of body fluid, or too little oxygen reaching the lungs.

Symptoms   Any or all of the following may be present:

1. Pale or bluish and cool skin.
2. Moist and clammy skin.
3. Overall weakness.
4. Rapid (over 100 beats per minute) and weak pulse.
5. Increased rate of breathing; shallow and irregular breathing or deep sighing.
6. Restlessness, anxiety.
7. Unusual thirst.
8. Vomiting.
9. Dull, sunken look to the eyes; pupils widely dilated.
10. Unresponsiveness.
11. Possible blotchy or streaked skin.
12. Possible unconsciousness in severe cases.

INJURIES AND ILLNESSES

Immediate
Treatment

1. Maintain an open airway.
2. Treat the cause of shock, such as breathing difficulties, bleeding, or severe pain.
3. Keep the victim lying down.
4. Cover the victim only enough to prevent loss of body heat. Keep him or her comfortable.
5. Seek medical attention promptly.
6. Check to see that the victim is not getting chilled. Keep him or her comfortably warm. If possible, place a blanket under a victim who is on the ground or on a damp surface.
7. Look for other injuries such as internal bleeding (see p. 85) and broken bones (see p. 93) and give first aid for those problems. This may decrease the severity of the shock.
8. *If medical attention is several hours away,* give the victim water or a weak solution of salt (1 level teaspoon) and baking soda (½ level teaspoon), mixed with 1 quart of cool water. Give an adult 4 ounces (½ glass); a child 1 to 12 years old 2 ounces; and an infant 1 ounce. Have the victim slip slowly over a 15-minute period. Fruit juices may also be given.

   Do not, however, give fluid if the victim is unconscious, having convulsions, likely to need surgery, has a brain injury, has a stomach wound, is vomiting, or is bleeding from the rectum. Stop fluids if vomiting occurs.
9. Reassure the victim. Gentleness, kindness, and understanding play an important role in treating a victim in shock.
10. If possible, obtain information about the nature of the accident.

Continued
Care

1. *Do not* move the victim if he or she has head, neck, or back injuries unless the victim is in danger of further injury. Maintain an open airway.
2. If the victim has no obvious injuries and the reason for shock is unknown, it is best to leave him or her lying flat.

3. Watch the victim very closely for changes in consciousness. Restore breathing and circulation if necessary.

INSULIN SHOCK

A specific type of shock occurs in individuals who have diabetes when there is too little blood sugar in the body. The condition arises when the victim takes too much insulin, or eats too little food after taking insulin or other diabetes medications.

Symptoms   Symptoms are *completely different* from those of a diabetic coma. Any or all of the following may be present:

1. Sudden onset.
2. Hunger, but no thirst.
3. Pale and sweaty skin.
4. Excited behavior and/or sometimes belligerent behavior.
5. Breath smells normal, not fruity.
6. Breathing is normal or shallow.
7. Mouth and tongue are moist.
8. No vomiting.

If the Victim Is **Conscious:**

Immediate   1. Give the victim food containing sugar, such as
Treatment   fruit juice, sweetened drinks, honey, or just sugar in water.
           2. Seek medical attention.

If the Victim Is **Unconscious:**

Seek medical attention promptly, preferably at the nearest hospital emergency room.

PSYCHOGENIC SHOCK

While shock in the true sense of the word does not occur, "psychogenic shock" is used to describe what happens to an individual who has experienced an overwhelming and psychologically stressful event, such as the death of a loved one or the crash of an airplane. These events may incapacitate the person.

Symptoms   Any or all of the following may be present:

1. Disorientation.
2. Inability to cope with the event.
3. Fainting.

What to Do   1. Stay with the victim.
2. Calm and reassure him or her.
3. Suggest that the victim seek medical treatment.

SEPTIC SHOCK

Septic shock—in which the body's tissues and vital organs are unable to use nutrients from the blood—is brought on by an infection in the bloodstream.

Symptoms   Any or all of the following may be present:

1. Sudden fever.
2. Vomiting.
3. Lightheadedness or dizziness.
4. Fainting.
5. Weakness.

Immediate   1. Maintain an open airway. Restore breathing
Treatment   (p. 20) and circulation (p. 22), if necessary.
2. Keep the victim lying down.
3. Cover the victim only enough to prevent loss of body heat. Keep the victim comfortable.
4. Seek medical attention promptly.

TOXIC SHOCK SYNDROME (TSS)

Toxic shock is a serious, but rare, medical condition caused by a bacterial staphylococcal infection. The infection usually is triggered by the use of high-absorbency tampons.

Toxins produced by the bacteria enter the bloodstream and are spread throughout the body. As in all cases of shock, toxic shock restricts the supply of oxygenated blood from reaching body tissues. *The condition can be fatal.*

Symptoms   Any or all of the following may be present:

1. Sudden fever.
2. Vomiting.
3. Lightheadedness or dizziness.
4. Fainting.
5. Weakness.
6. Rash, similar to a sunburn, that may spread to the palms of the hands and soles of the feet.

Immediate   1. Maintain an open airway. Restore breathing
Treatment   (p. 20) and circulation (p. 22), if necessary.
             2. Keep the victim lying down.
             3. Cover the victim only enough to prevent loss of body heat. Keep the victim comfortable.
             4. If a tampon has been inserted, remove it.
             5. Seek medical attention promptly.

See Also: Bites and Stings (Insect Stings), p. 64; Bleeding, p. 80; Convulsions, p. 133; Drug Abuse, p. 154; Electric Shock, p. 166; Heart Attack, p. 196; Unconsciousness, p. 251; Wounds, p. 257.

INJURIES AND ILLNESSES

SPLINTERS

A splinter, or sliver, is a small piece of wood, glass, or other material that becomes lodged under the surface of the skin.

What to Do

1. Wash your hands and the victim's skin around the splinter with soap and water.
2. Place a sewing needle and tweezers in boiling water for about 5 minutes or hold over an open flame to sterilize.
3. If the splinter is sticking out of the skin, gently pull the splinter out with the tweezers at the same angle at which it entered.
4. If the splinter is not deeply lodged below the skin and is clearly visible, gently loosen the skin around the splinter with the needle and carefully remove the splinter with the tweezers at the same angle at which it entered.
5. Squeeze the wound gently to allow slight bleeding to wash out germs. Or wash out the wound under running water.
6. If the splinter breaks off in the skin or is deeply lodged, seek medical attention for removal and possible tetanus shot.
7. After the splinter is removed, wash the area with soap and water and apply a bandage.
8. Watch for any signs of infection such as redness, pus, or red streaks leading up the body from the wound.

See Also: Bleeding, p. 80.

SPRAINS

A sprain is an injury to the ligaments, which support the joints in the body. The ligaments may be stretched or completely torn. A sprain usually results from overextending or twisting a limb beyond its normal range of movement, thus stretching and tearing some of the fibers of the ligament.

Symptoms
1. Pain upon moving the injured part. Pain in the joint.
2. Swelling of the joint.
3. Tenderness upon touching the affected area.
4. Black and blue discoloration of skin around the area of the injury.

What to Do
If uncertain as to whether the injury is a sprain or a broken bone, treat as a broken bone. (See Broken Bones, p. 93.)

If the Ankle *or* Knee *Is Sprained:*

1. Place cold wet packs or a small ice bag wrapped in a cloth over the affected area intermittently for the first 12 to 24 hours to decrease swelling.
2. Apply supporting bandage, pillow, or blanket splint. (See Splinting and Other Procedures, p. 95.) Loosen support if swelling increases.
3. Keep the injured part elevated above the level of the heart.
4. Keep the victim from walking, if possible.
5. *Do not* use heat or hot water soaks immediately following the injury. They may be applied intermittently not less than 24 hours after the injury.
6. It is best to seek medical attention to rule out a broken bone. Always seek medical attention if pain or swelling persists.

If the Wrist, Elbow, *or* Shoulder *Is Sprained:*

What to Do
1. Place the injured arm in a sling. (See Bandages, p. 42.)
2. Place cold wet packs or a small ice bag wrapped in a cloth over the affected area. *Do not* use heat or hot water soaks immediately following the injury.
3. For a wrist injury, apply a supporting bandage. Loosen the bandage if swelling increases.
4. It is best to seek medical attention to rule out a broken bone. Always seek medical attention if pain or swelling persists.

See Also: Broken Bones and Spinal Injuries, p. 93; Dislocations, p. 147; Muscle Aches and Pains, p. 208; Part III: Sports First Aid, pp. 267–319.

STRAINS

A strain results from pulling or overexerting a muscle. Back strains are common injuries.

What to Do
1. Rest the affected area immediately.
2. Apply ice or a cold compress to the affected area to decrease swelling.
3. After 24 hours, apply warm wet compresses to the affected area.
4. If possible, elevate the strained area.
5. Seek medical attention if pain or swelling is severe.

See Also: Muscle Aches and Pains, p. 208; Part III: Sports First Aid, pp. 267–319.

INJURIES AND ILLNESSES

STROKE

A stroke can be a life-threatening situation. It usually occurs when there is an interruption of the blood supply to part or all of the brain. This interruption in circulation may be caused by the formation of a clot inside an artery supplying blood to the brain, by a clot from elsewhere in the body that blocks blood supply to the brain, by the narrowing of a blood vessel, or by the bursting of an artery within the brain. The brain must receive adequate amounts of blood to function properly.

ABCs

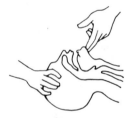

With all serious injuries, check and maintain an open airway. Restore breathing (p. 20) and circulation (p. 22), if necessary.

MAJOR STROKE

Symptoms   Any or all of the following may be present:

1. Sudden headache.
2. Sudden paralysis, weakness, or numbness of the face, arm, or leg on one side of the body. The corner of the mouth may droop.
3. Loss or slurring of speech.
4. Possible unconsciousness or mental confusion.
5. Sudden fall.
6. Impaired vision.
7. Pupils of the eyes different in size.

8. Difficulty with breathing, chewing, talking, and/or swallowing.
9. Loss of bladder and/or bowel control.
10. Strong, slow pulse.

Immediate 1. Seek medical attention promptly.
Treatment 2. Maintain an open airway.
3. Restore breathing if necessary, p. 20.

Mouth-to-Mouth Resuscitation

If the Victim Is Not Breathing:

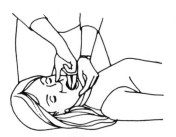

1. Make sure the victim is on a hard, flat surface. Quickly clear the mouth and airway of foreign material.

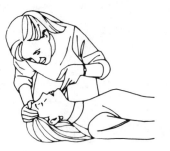

2. Tilt the victim's head backward by placing the palm of your hand on his or her forehead and the fingers of your other hand under the bony part of the chin.

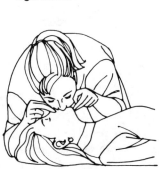

3. Pinch the victim's nostrils with your thumb and index finger. Take a deep breath. Place your mouth tightly over the victim's mouth (mouth and nose for an infant or small child). Give 2 quick breaths.

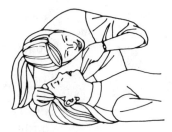

4. Stop blowing when the chest is expanding. Remove your mouth from the victim's mouth and turn your head toward the victim's chest, so that your ear is over his or her mouth. *Listen* for air being exhaled. *Watch* for the victim's chest to fall. Repeat the breathing procedure.

Continued Care

1. Place the victim on his or her weak side so that secretions can drain from the mouth.
2. Keep the victim comfortably warm.
3. Keep the victim quiet.
4. Apply cold cloths to the victim's head.
5. Reassure and calm the victim.
6. *Do not* give fluids or food to the victim. He or she may vomit or choke on them.

MINOR STROKE

Symptoms

1. Slight mental confusion.
2. Slight dizziness.
3. Minor speech difficulties.
4. Muscle weakness.

What to Do   Seek medical attention.

TRANSIENT ISCHEMIC ATTACK (TIA)

A transient ischemic attack (TIA) is a spasm of a cerebral (brain) blood vessel. Symptoms usually occur in individuals between the ages of 50 and 70 and usually clear up within 24 hours.

Symptoms   Any or all of the following may be present:

1. Slight mental confusion.
2. Slight dizziness.
3. Minor speech difficulties.
4. Muscle weakness.

What to Do   Seek medical care as soon as possible for further evaluation and to prevent more serious problems from arising.

SUICIDE, THREATENED

All threats of suicide must be taken seriously. The person threatening to take his or her life sees the situation as hopeless and sees death as the answer to problems. Yet most victims need and want help. The victim may very well change his or her mind if given the chance to do so and it is that chance you want to provide by diverting the immediate thoughts of self-destruction.

If the threat of suicide is unmistakable—that is, the victim is holding a gun, knife, or bottle of pills—you must get the situation under control immediately. Remain calm. Call the police or other professionals trained in dealing with crisis situations. Do not show anger toward the victim or argue with him or her. Speak in a soft tone and do not make any sudden movement. What you want to do is provide *time*. Encourage the victim to talk, and listen attentively. Express interest and concern in what the victim is saying. Once the immediate self-destruction situation is under control, seek professional help for the victim. If possible, go with the victim, as he or she needs to know that someone cares.

If the victim is talking about suicide but does not have the means at hand, the immediate situation is not as critical, although *all* suicide talk must be taken seriously. Talk with the victim if he or she is willing to do so. Listen attentively and express interest in and concern about the situation. Do not pressure the victim into talking if he or she does not wish to talk. Always seek professional help when someone expresses a wish to die.

Suicide threats among children are *very* serious, and a child talking of suicide should *not* be left alone until a thorough psychiatric evaluation is done.

There are certain clues and symptoms that may indicate that a person is thinking of suicide. One of these symptoms is severe de-

249

pression. This is not the same as occasional depressed moods that last only a few days. The victim of severe depression suffers a loss of appetite, loss of sleep, and sees no joy or pleasure in his or her life over a long period of time. Other danger signs include heavy drinking of alcoholic beverages, previous threats or attempts at suicide, a history of suicide in the victim's family, giving away or selling valuable possessions, recent filing of a will, or not renewing a rental lease.

See Also: Drug Abuse, p. 154.

UNCONSCIOUSNESS

There are many causes of unconsciousness. Among these are heart attack, stroke, head injury, bleeding, diabetic coma, insulin shock, poisoning, heatstroke, choking, gas inhalation, severe allergic reaction to insect stings, and electric shock.

Symptoms
1. Unresponsiveness.
2. Unawareness of surroundings.

(If the victim is breathing, see p. 253.)

*If the Unconscious Victim Is **Not** Breathing:*

ABCs

With all serious injuries, check and maintain an open airway. Restore breathing (p. 20) and circulation (p. 22), if necessary.

Immediate
Treatment
1. Restore breathing (p. 20) and circulation (p. 22), if necessary.

(*continued on p. 253*)

INJURIES AND ILLNESSES

Mouth-to-Mouth Resuscitation

If the victim is not breathing and no neck injury is suspected, perform all of the following 4 steps.

If a neck injury is suspected (as in a diving or motorcycle accident, or from a fall from a height) *do not* twist or rotate the head. Slightly elevate the chin only to open the airway. Check for foreign material in the mouth. Then continue with steps 3 and 4, below.*

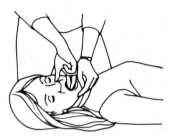

1. Make sure the victim is on a hard, flat surface. Quickly clear the mouth and airway of foreign material.

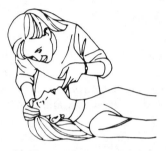

2. Tilt the victim's head backward by placing the palm of your hand on his or her forehead and the fingers of your other hand under the bony part of the chin.

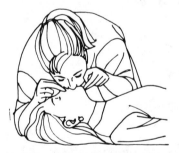

3. Pinch the victim's nostrils with your thumb and index finger. Take a deep breath. Place your mouth tightly over the victim's mouth (mouth and nose for an infant or small child). Give 2 quick breaths.

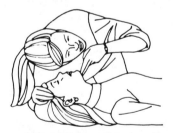

4. Stop blowing when the chest is expanding. Remove your mouth from the victim's mouth and turn your head toward the victim's chest, so that your ear is over his or her mouth. *Listen* for air being exhaled. *Watch* for the victim's chest to fall. Repeat the breathing procedure.

*To move a victim with a neck injury, see p. 191.

(*continued from p. 251*)
If the Unconscious Victim **Is** *Breathing from Onset:*

Immediate
Treatment

1. Maintain an open airway.
2. Loosen tight clothing, particularly around the victim's neck.
3. Keep the victim lying down. If the cause of unconsciousness is unknown, always suspect a head, neck, or back injury and do not move the victim except to maintain an open airway. If the cause of unconsciousness is known, such as heatstroke (p. 210) or diabetic coma (p. 142), place the victim on his or her side to allow secretions to drain and to prevent choking on fluids and vomit. When placed on his or her side, the victim should have the head slightly lower than the rest of the body.
4. Check for possible cause of unconsciousness, such as bleeding (p. 80), broken bones (p. 93), or a head injury (p. 188), and give first aid. *Do not* waste time treating minor injuries.
5. Seek medical attention promptly, preferably at the nearest hospital emergency room.

Continued
Care

1. Keep the victim comfortably warm but not hot.
2. *Do not* give an unconscious victim anything to eat or drink.
3. *Do not* leave an unconscious victim alone.

INJURIES AND ILLNESSES

VERTIGO

Vertigo is a disturbance in the balance mechanism of the inner ear. This disturbance may be caused by an ear infection, an allergy, injury to the inner ear, or from decreased blood flow to the head.

Symptoms   Any or all of the following may be present:

1. Loss of balance.
2. Dizziness (feeling that everything is spinning around or that the victim is spinning around).
3. Nausea with or without vomiting.

What to Do
1. Reassure the victim that he or she is not turning or spinning around.
2. Assist the victim so that he or she does not fall.
3. Seek medical attention.

VOMITING

Vomiting may occur with many conditions. It is particularly common with viral infections of the intestines, excessive eating, excessive drinking of alcoholic beverages, and emotional upsets.

Vomiting may be present with more serious conditions such as appendicitis, bowel obstruction, asthma, animal bites, allergic reactions to insect stings, black widow or brown recluse spider bites, marine life bites, scorpion bites, poisonous snake bites, withdrawal from drugs, heart attack, heat exhaustion, shock due to injuries, diabetic coma, food poisoning, and head injuries.

Vomiting associated with intestinal viruses, excessive eating or drinking, and emotional stress usually does not last a long time. Any vomiting, however, that is severe or lasts longer than a day or two needs medical attention, as dehydration (loss of body fluids) or a chemical imbalance (loss of body chemicals) can occur. This is especially true in infants, the elderly, or chronically ill persons.

Vomiting can indicate a serious problem. Seek medical attention promptly if vomiting occurs with severe stomach pain or after a recent head injury, or if the vomit contains blood that looks like coffee grounds.

What to Do
In treatment of simple vomiting associated with intestinal upsets, replace lost fluids by frequent sipping of liquids such as carbonated beverages (shaken up to eliminate fizz), tea, juice, or bouillon. After vomiting has stopped, avoid solid food. Work slowly back to a regular diet.

If the victim is unconscious and vomiting, he or she should be placed on his or her side with the head extended, as long as there is no head, neck, or back injury. Doing this will prevent the victim from choking on the vomit. A victim with a head injury should have his or her head turned to the side to prevent choking.

VOMITING IN INFANTS AND YOUNG CHILDREN

Vomiting in infants and children is common. Some of the most common causes include allergy, viral infections (flu), poisoning, car sickness, intestinal obstructions, pneumonia, colic, head injuries, nerves, and appendicitis.

In newborns and infants, spitting up food after eating is common and is *not* the same as vomiting. It is usually not serious. Be sure the infant does not choke.

Vomiting in infants can be quite serious, particularly if vomited material is expelled with such force that it shoots out of the infant's mouth 1 or 2 feet across the room (projectile vomiting). This type of vomiting always needs prompt medical attention. It could represent a partially or completely obstructed intestine.

Prolonged vomiting or vomiting with diarrhea can lead to dehydration (loss of body fluids) and also needs prompt medical attention.

Other possibly serious symptoms to watch for in infants and small children include vomit that contains blood, and vomiting with headaches or stomachaches.

What to Do   In treatment of simple vomiting that accompanies intestinal upsets, for example, the victim should drink fluids and avoid solid foods. Give him or her small sips (approximately 1 teaspoon) of carbonated beverages (shaken up to eliminate fizz), tea, or juice (not orange) every 10 to 20 minutes. Gradually increase amount if victim keeps fluids down. Slowly work back to a regular diet once the stomach is settled.

See Also: Abdominal Pain in Infants and Children, p. 57; Bites and Stings, p. 63; Diarrhea, p. 144; Drug Abuse, p. 154; Food Poisoning, p. 183; Overexposure: Heat and Cold, p. 209.

WOUNDS

OPEN WOUNDS

An open wound is an injury in which the skin is broken. The objectives in treating an open wound consist of:

1. Stopping the bleeding.
2. Preventing contamination and infection.
3. Preventing or treating for shock if necessary.
4. Seeking medical attention if the wound is severe or if the victim has not had a tetanus shot within 5 to 7 years.

Abdominal Wounds

Deep abdominal wounds are an emergency. Surgery will probably be necessary to repair the wound.

ABCs

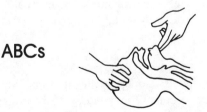

With all serious injuries, check and maintain an open *a*irway. Restore *b*reathing (p. 20) and *c*irculation (p. 22), if necessary.

Immediate Treatment

1. Maintain an open airway and restore breathing if necessary, p. 20.
2. Keep the victim lying down on his or her back.

3. Bend the victim's legs at the knees and place a pillow, a rolled towel, a blanket, or clothing under the knees to relax the abdominal muscles.

4. Apply direct pressure if necessary to control bleeding. (See Bleeding [Internal Bleeding], p. 85.) The abdomen is soft and pressure decreases or stops internal bleeding.

5. *Do not* try to push intestines back in place if they are sticking out of the wound.

6. If medical assistance is not readily available and the intestine is sticking out of the wound, dampen a pad with sterile or boiled and *then cooled* water, if available. Drinking water or clean seawater may be used in an emergency. Place this damp pad over the intestine.

7. Cover the *entire* wound with a sterile pad such as gauze (preferably) or a clean cloth, clothing, towel, plastic wrap, aluminum foil, or other suitable material.

8. Apply a firm bandage to hold the pad in place. Do not bandage too tightly.

9. Keep the victim comfortably warm.

10. *Do not* give the victim anything to eat or drink, including water, as surgery will probably be necessary and the stomach should be empty.

11. Seek medical attention immediately at the nearest hospital emergency room.

Chest Wounds

In a deep open chest wound, damage to the lungs may occur, resulting in air flowing in and out of the wound with breathing and not in and out of the lungs, where it is needed. This is a serious emergency.

Immediate Treatment

1. *Do not* remove any object remaining in the wound, as *very* serious bleeding or other internal life-threatening problems may result.

(*continued on p. 260*)

Mouth-to-Mouth Resuscitation

If the victim is not breathing and no neck injury is suspected, perform all of the following 4 steps.

If a neck injury is suspected (as in a diving or motorcycle accident, or from a fall from a height) *do not* twist or rotate the head. *Slightly* elevate the chin only to open the airway. Check for foreign material in the mouth. Then continue with steps 3 and 4, below.*

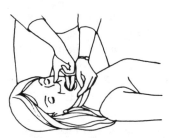

1. Make sure the victim is on a hard, flat surface. Quickly clear the mouth and airway of foreign material.

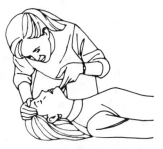

2. Tilt the victim's head backward by placing the palm of your hand on his or her forehead and the fingers of your other hand under the bony part of the chin.

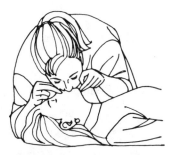

3. Pinch the victim's nostrils with your thumb and index finger. Take a deep breath. Place your mouth tightly over the victim's mouth (mouth and nose for an infant or small child). Give 2 quick breaths.

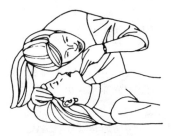

4. Stop blowing when the chest is expanding. Remove your mouth from the victim's mouth and turn your head toward the victim's chest, so that your ear is over his or her mouth. *Listen* for air being exhaled. *Watch* for the victim's chest to fall. Repeat the breathing procedure.

*To move a victim with a neck injury, see p. 191.

INJURIES AND ILLNESSES

(*continued from p. 258*)

2. Immediately cover the *entire* wound with a pad, such as dry sterile gauze (preferably), a clean cloth, clothing, plastic wrap, aluminum foil, or other suitable material. The pad *must* be large enough to cover the entire wound and must be airtight so that air will not escape.

3. If no pad is available, place a hand on each side of the wound and firmly push the skin together to close the wound.

4. Apply an airtight bandage with tape or other suitable material if available.

5. Maintain an open airway and restore breathing if necessary, p. 20.

6. Treat the victim for shock (p. 234). It may be necessary to slightly raise the victim's shoulders to aid breathing.

7. *Do not* give the victim anything to eat or drink, as this may cause choking. Also, the stomach should be empty in case surgery is necessary.

8. Reassure the victim. Gentleness, kindness, and understanding play an important role in treating a victim in shock.

9. Seek medical attention immediately at the nearest hospital emergency room.

Cuts (Lacerations)

If Bleeding Is Severe:

Immediate Treatment   Use direct pressure to control bleeding. (See Bleeding [External Bleeding], p. 80.)

If Bleeding Is Not *Severe:*

What to Do
1. Wash your hands thoroughly with soap and water before handling the wound to prevent further contamination of the injury.

2. If the cut is still bleeding, apply direct pressure over the wound with a sterile or clean cloth.

3. When the bleeding has stopped, wash the wound thoroughly with soap and water to

remove any dirt or other foreign material near the skin's surface. Gentle scrubbing may be necessary. It is very important to remove all dirt to prevent infection. Foreign particles close to the skin's surface may be carefully removed with tweezers that have been sterilized over an open flame or boiled in water.

4. *Do not* attempt to remove any foreign material that is deeply embedded in a muscle or other tissue, as serious bleeding may result. This must be done by a doctor.

5. Rinse the wound thoroughly under running water.

6. Pat the wound dry with a sterile or clean cloth.

7. *Do not* apply ointments, medication, antiseptic spray, or home remedies unless told to do so by a doctor.

8. Cover the wound with a sterile dressing and bandage it in place. If the cut is slightly gaping, apply a butterfly bandage (see p. 42) or tape the wound to get the edges as close together as possible.

9. Always seek medical attention if:
    (a) The wound is severe.
    (b) The bleeding does not stop.
    (c) The injury was caused by an obviously dirty object.
    (d) A foreign material or object is embedded in the wound.
    (e) Signs of infection such as fever, redness, swelling, increased tenderness at the site of the wound, pus, or red streaks leading from the wound toward the body appear.
    (f) There is any doubt about tetanus immunization.

10. If medical assistance is not readily available and the wound shows signs of infection, keep the victim lying down with the injured area immobilized and elevated. Apply warm wet cloths over the wound until medical assistance can be obtained.

INJURIES AND ILLNESSES

Puncture Wounds

A puncture wound results from a sharp object, such as a nail, a large splinter, a knife, a needle, a bullet, a firecracker, or an ice pick, piercing the skin and the underlying tissue. The wound is usually deep and narrow, with little bleeding. This increases the chance for infection because the germs are not washed out by the flow of blood.

Tetanus is a danger with any wound, but is greater with puncture wounds since the tetanus bacteria grow well in a deep wound where there is little oxygen. *All* puncture injuries should be seen by a doctor.

What to Do
1. Wash your hands with soap and water before examining the wound.
2. Look to see if any part of the offending object has broken off and become lodged in the wound.
3. *Do not* attempt to remove any foreign object that is deeply embedded in the wound, as the foreign object may break off in the wound and/or serious bleeding may result. This must be done by a doctor.
4. *Do not* poke or put medication into the wound.
5. In obviously minor puncture wounds, objects sticking in no deeper than the skin's surface may be carefully removed with tweezers that have been sterilized over an open flame or boiled in water.
6. Encourage bleeding to wash out germs from inside the wound by gently pressing on the edge of the wound.
   Do not press so hard as to cause additional injury to the wound.
7. If the puncture wound is obviously minor, wash the wound with soap and water and rinse under running water.
8. Cover the wound with a sterile or clean dressing and bandage in place.
9. Treat for shock if necessary. (See Shock, p. 234.)

10. Seek medical attention promptly.
11. If medical attention is not readily available and the wound shows signs of infection such as fever, redness, swelling, increased tenderness at the site of the wound, pus, or red streaks leading from the wound toward the body, keep the victim lying down with the injured area immobilized and elevated. Apply warm wet cloths over the wound until medical assistance can be obtained.

Scrapes and Scratches

Scrapes can become easily infected since the outer protective skin layer is destroyed in the scraped area.

What to Do
1. Wash your hands with soap and water before treating the wound.
2. Wash the injured area well with soap and water to remove any dirt. Gentle scrubbing may be necessary. It is important to remove all dirt to prevent infection. Bits of dirt left in the wound may also cause permanent discoloration of the skin. Rinse the wound under running water.
3. *Do not* put medication on the wound unless so directed by a doctor.
4. Minor scrapes and scratches can be left exposed to the air. Cover larger wounds, or those likely to be reinjured, with a sterile pad or clean cloth and bandage in place.
5. Watch for signs of infection. If the wound shows signs of infection, such as redness, swelling, increased tenderness at the site of the wound, pus, or red streaks leading from the wound toward the body, keep the victim lying down, with the injured area immobilized and elevated. Apply warm wet cloths over the wound until medical assistance can be obtained.
6. Also seek medical attention if the wound is large or deep or there is a question of tetanus immunization.

CLOSED WOUNDS

Closed wounds are not always obvious, as there is no break in the skin. Suspect internal wounds if the victim has been in an accident, fallen, or received a severe body blow to the chest, abdomen, head, or spine. Internal injuries may be very serious.

Symptoms   Any or all of the following may be present:

1. Pain and tenderness at the site of the injury. Redness of the skin where blow occurred.
2. Vomit that resembles coffee grounds.
3. Coughed-up blood that is bright red.
4. Stools containing dark, tarry material or bright red blood.
5. Urine containing blood.
6. Pale skin.
7. Cold, clammy skin.
8. Rapid but weak pulse.
9. Rapid breathing.
10. Dizziness.
11. Swelling.
12. Restlessness.
13. Thirst.

Immediate Treatment
1. Maintain an open airway and restore breathing if necessary, p. 20.
2. Seek medical attention promptly.

Continued Care
1. Keep the victim lying down and quiet.
2. If the victim is vomiting, turn his or her head to the side to prevent choking.
3. If the victim has difficulty breathing, raise his or her shoulders with a pillow.
4. Check for other injuries, such as broken bones (See Broken Bones and Spinal Injuries, p. 93.)
5. Keep the victim comfortably warm.
6. *Do not* give the victim anything to eat or drink, including water.
7. Reassure the victim. Gentleness, kindness, and understanding play an important role in treating a victim of any injury or illness.
8. If the victim must be moved by someone other than trained medical personnel, keep the victim lying down and be very careful.

See Also: Bleeding, p. 80; Broken Bones and Spinal Injuries, p. 93; Head and Neck Injuries, p. 188; Shock, p. 234.

PART III

SPORTS
FIRST AID

BACK

Low Back Pain

What the Lower Back Is: The lower back consists of the vertebrae and discs of the lumbar spine; the sacrum and coccyx (tailbone) of the lower back; and many muscle groups and ligaments that connect the chest wall to the pelvis.

What the Back Does: The spine and muscles provide support for the trunk of the body and protect the spinal cord.

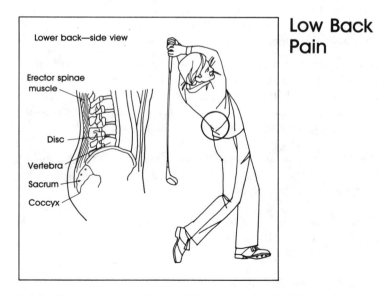

Lower back—side view

Erector spinae muscle

Disc

Vertebra

Sacrum

Coccyx

Low Back Pain

Low back pain can occur for a variety of reasons: a strain or tear in a muscle or ligament, injury to a disc or vertebra, pressure on a nerve, or fatigue.

What the Injury Is: Lower back pain in sports can occur for a variety of reasons: a strain or tear in a muscle or ligament; injury to a disc or vertebra; pressure on a nerve; or fatigue.

Cause: The injury can be caused by a repetitive motion over time, as in the golf swing, for example, or by a sudden force exerted on the back, as in a football block. It can also occur because of an insufficient warm-up period prior to athletic activity.

Symptoms: Anything from a dull ache to a sharp pain in the lower back. If a muscle tears, you may feel a slight pull when the injury occurs, with pain intensifying several hours after the injury. A herniated disc may produce sharp pains that makes any movement impossible. Sciatic nerve damage may produce sharp pains that radiate down the back of one or both legs. A back that is fatigued, from a long-distance sports event, for example, may be stiff and ache all over.

Immediate Treatment: *See your physician without delay if pain is severe or radiates down the back of both legs, if numbness or tingling is present in the lower back and legs, or if bowel or bladder abnormalities occur.*

For Muscle Pulls or Tears: Place an ice pack on the back as soon as possible after the injury occurs. *Cold* treatments help stop internal bleeding and the accumulation of fluids in and around the injured area, thus decreasing swelling.

For Stiffness or Fatigue: Place a heating pad on the back to help relax the muscles. Soreness in the lower back can also be relieved by lying down, which takes the pressure of gravity off the back; by placing one foot on a foot rest, which shifts the angle of the sacrum, thus lessening the arch of the back; or by a good night's rest.

Medication: (If you have seen your physician, follow his or her advice.) Take aspirin, ibuprofen, or acetaminophen regularly to relieve pain and inflammation.

NOTE: *Acetaminophen may not contain as much of the anti-inflammatory agents as aspirin or ibuprofen. Ask your physician or pharmacist for guidance.*

WARNING: *Do not give aspirin to children under the age of 16. If pregnant or nursing, consult with your physician first before taking any medication.*

Continued Care:

For Muscle Pulls or Tears: Use an ice pack on the injury at least once a day for 2 to 4 days. Thereafter, use a heating pad on the back at least once a day until the injury heals. *Heat* treatments help to enlarge the small blood vessels in and around the injured area, thus increasing blood circulation. (Blood carries vital nutrients to the injury and helps speed recovery.)

NOTE: *Heat should be applied only after the swelling has stopped, or swelling in the injured area may increase.*

Avoid athletic activity until the injury has had time to heal or until there is no pain in the back. The length of time for the injury to heal, depending upon the type and severity of the injury, may be 3 to 6 weeks, or longer. Once the injury has healed, gradually and carefully perform exercises that stretch the muscles in the back. Use an ice pack to reduce any swelling that may occur, then heat—after swelling has subsided—to help relax the muscles.

For Stiffness or Fatigue: See information under Immediate Treatment, above.

Medication: Take aspirin, ibuprofen, or acetaminophen to relieve pain and inflammation.

Long-Term Effects of Injury: None, with proper rest.

Prevention of Recurring Injury: Work with a trainer or physical therapist on exercises that strengthen the back and abdominal muscles. Stretch the muscles in the back before engaging in sports. Avoid sudden movements that could reinjure the back.

See Your Physician: If pain continues or reinjury occurs.

SPORTS FIRST AID

ELBOW

Golfer's Elbow

What the Elbow Is: The elbow consists of three main bones—the humerus of the upper arm and the ulna and radius of the forearm (lower arm)—that converge to form the elbow joint. The bony protrusions on the inside and outside of the elbow are called epicondyles. Ligaments—connective tissue—connect the three bones in the elbow. Tendons—also connective tissue—connect muscles to the

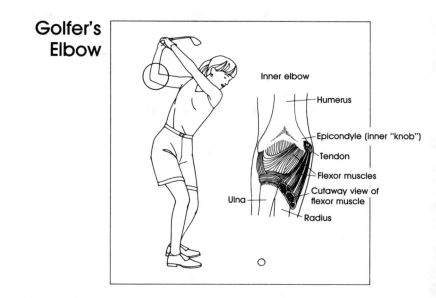

Golfer's Elbow

Inner elbow
Humerus
Epicondyle (inner "knob")
Tendon
Flexor muscles
Cutaway view of flexor muscle
Ulna
Radius

Golfer's elbow is tendinitis in the tendon that attaches the flexor muscles to the inner "knob" of the elbow.

270

bones. Bursas—fluid-filled sacs or saclike cavities—surround and cushion these bones at the joint.

What the Elbow Does: The elbow is a hinge joint that allows rotation of the wrist and hand, and extension and flexion of the forearm.

What the Injury Is: Golfer's elbow, the opposite of tennis elbow, is an inflammation or microtear in the tendon (tendinitis) that attaches the flexor muscle group to the medial (inside) epicondyle. The flexor group of muscles runs down the inside of the forearm and helps to flex (bend) the wrist and to close the fingers.

Cause: Commonly seen in both tennis players and golfers, the injury is usually associated with a repetitive motion over time. It can develop from an improper downward stroke in golf or hitting the ground repetitively during the golf swing; from an improperly executed forehand stroke in tennis; or from underdeveloped flexor muscles. Other sports that can cause golfer's elbow: racquetball, paddle tennis, rowing, bowling, archery, waterskiing, and weight lifting. Other activities that may cause golfer's elbow: construction work and other kinds of manual labor (such as housework, moving furniture, or mopping floors), painting, and gardening.

Symptoms: Pain on the inside of the elbow. The pain can be intense and limit movement. It can be present, for example, when picking up children, carrying a heavy tray, or lifting boxes.

Immediate Treatment: *Always, in serious cases of golfer's elbow, such as when the elbow cannot be bent or straightened without pain, see your physician to determine proper treatment.* Stop the activity that is causing the pain. Place an ice pack on the elbow as soon as possible. *Cold* treatments help stop internal bleeding and the accumulation of fluids in and around the injured area, thus decreasing swelling.

Medication: (If you have seen your physician, follow his or her advice.) Take aspirin, ibuprofen, or acetaminophen regularly to relieve pain and inflammation. Your physician may prescribe another mild analgesic (pain reliever) to help reduce pain or a nonsteroidal anti-inflammatory drug (NSAID) to help reduce pain and swelling. In some instances, your physician may suggest a low-dose injection of a corticosteroid or "steroid" drug, such as cortisone, that will help to reduce inflammation.

SPORTS FIRST AID

NOTE: *Acetaminophen may not contain as much of the anti-inflammatory agents as aspirin or ibuprofen. Ask your physician or pharmacist for guidance.*

WARNING: *Do not give aspirin to children under the age of 16. If pregnant or nursing, consult with your physician first before taking any medication.*

Continued Care: Rest the arm for 4 to 8 weeks. Use an ice pack at least once a day for 2 to 4 days after ceasing the activity to reduce swelling and inflammation. Use a heating pad thereafter. *Heat* treatments help to enlarge the small blood vessels in and around the injured area, thus increasing blood circulation. (Blood carries vital nutrients to the injury and helps speed recovery.)

NOTE: *Heat should be applied only after swelling has abated, or swelling in the injured area may increase.*

Do not engage in original activity until the pain has subsided. Ease into limited muscle workouts: swing a golf club or tennis racquet, work with light weights, and work with a trainer or physical therapist for hand, wrist, and forearm exercises that use and strengthen the flexor muscles. Muscle-strengthening exercises also help strengthen ligaments and tendons. Use an ice pack first to reduce swelling, then a heating pad to aid recovery.

Medication: Take aspirin, ibuprofen, or acetaminophen to help reduce pain and inflammation.

Long-Term Effects of Injury: None, with proper treatment and rest, although some individuals may suffer recurring tendinitis even with precautionary measures (see below). In rare cases, surgery to release tension on the tendon, which involves severing the tendon from the bone, may be recommended.

Prevention of Recurring Injury. Allow plenty of time for healing. Use weights and exercises advised by a trainer or physical therapist. These measures may have to be employed throughout a lifetime to avoid or reduce pain. Obtain the advice of a golf or tennis pro on proper equipment and technique. Wear a tennis strap or band just below the elbow. The strap helps to constrict both the extensor and flexor muscles and takes the pressure off the areas at which the muscles attach to the elbow (lateral and medial epicondyles). This measure alone may greatly reduce pain. Use an ice pack first to reduce swelling, then a heating pad to aid recovery.

See Your Physician: If pain is severe and limits flexion (bending) of the arm.

Tennis Elbow

What the Elbow Is: The elbow consists of three main bones—the humerus of the upper arm and the ulna and radius of the forearm (lower arm)—that converge to form the elbow joint. The bony protrusions on the inside and outside of the elbow are called epicondyles. Ligaments—connective tissue—connect the three bones in the elbow. Tendons—also connective tissue—connect muscles to the bones. Bursas—fluid-filled sacs or saclike cavities—surround and cushion these bones at the joint.

What the Elbow Does: The elbow is a hinge joint that allows rotation of the wrist and hand, and extension and flexion of the forearm.

What the Injury Is: Tennis elbow is a catchall phrase for an inflammation or microtear in the tendon (tendinitis) that connects

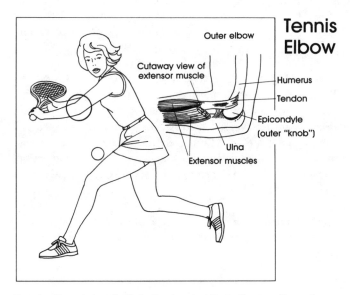

Tennis Elbow

Outer elbow

Cutaway view of extensor muscle

Humerus

Tendon

Epicondyle (outer "knob")

Ulna

Extensor muscles

Tennis elbow is tendinitis in the tendon that attaches the extensor muscles to the outer "knob" of the elbow.

SPORTS FIRST AID

the extensor muscle group to the lateral (outside) epicondyle. This group of muscles—the long muscles on the outside of the forearm—helps to open and extend the hand.

Cause: The injury is usually associated with a repetitive motion over time. Commonly, in tennis, it develops from an improperly executed backhand stroke. It may also be caused by improper equipment: a racquet that is too stiff or too heavy, a grip that is too small or too large, or strings that are too loose. Other causes: the wrist snap on the tennis serve and underdeveloped extensor muscles. Other sports that can cause tennis elbow: racquetball, paddle tennis, bowling, fly fishing, archery, skiing, and golf. Other activities that may cause tennis elbow: construction work and other kinds of manual labor (such as housework), painting, writing, and gardening.

Symptoms: Pain on the outside of the elbow. The pain can be severe and limit movement. Shaking hands, holding a coffee cup, turning a doorknob, or picking up a piece of paper may all produce extreme pain.

Immediate Treatment: *Always, in serious cases of tennis elbow, such as when the arm cannot be extended forward (as in a handshake), see your physician to determine proper treatment.* Stop the activity that is causing the pain. Place an ice pack on the elbow as soon as possible. *Cold* treatments help stop internal bleeding and the accumulation of fluids in and around the injured area, thus decreasing swelling.

Medication: (If you have seen your physician, follow his or her advice.) Take aspirin, ibuprofen, or acetaminophen regularly to relieve pain and inflammation. Your physician may prescribe another mild analgesic (pain reliever) to help reduce pain or a nonsteroidal anti-inflammatory drug (NSAID) to help reduce pain and swelling. In some instances, your physician may suggest a low-dose injection of a corticosteroid or "steroid" drug, such as cortisone, that will help to reduce inflammation.

NOTE: *Acetaminophen may not contain as much of the anti-inflammatory agents as aspirin or ibuprofen. Ask your physician or pharmacist for guidance.*

WARNING: *Do not give aspirin to children under the age of 16. If pregnant or nursing, consult with your physician first before taking any medication.*

Continued Care: Rest the arm for approximately 4 to 8 weeks. Use an ice pack at least once a day for 2 to 4 days after ceasing the activity, to reduce swelling and inflammation. Use a heating pad thereafter. *Heat* treatments help to enlarge the small blood vessels in and around the injured area, thus increasing blood circulation. (Blood carries vital nutrients to the injury and helps speed recovery.)

NOTE: *Heat should be applied only after swelling has subsided, or swelling in the injured area may increase.*

Do not engage in original activity until the pain has subsided. Ease into limited muscle workouts: swing a racquet, work with light weights, and work with a trainer or physical therapist for hand, wrist, and forearm exercises that use and strengthen the extensor muscles. Muscle-strengthening exercises also help strengthen ligaments and tendons. Use an ice pack first to reduce swelling, then a heating pad to aid recovery.

Medication: Take aspirin, ibuprofen, or acetaminophen to relieve pain and inflammation.

Long-Term Effects of Injury: None, with proper treatment and rest, although some individuals may suffer recurring tendinitis even with precautionary measures (see below). In rare cases, surgery to release tension on the tendon, which involves severing the tendon from the bone, may be recommended.

Prevention of Recurring Injury: Allow plenty of time for healing. Use weights and exercises advised by a trainer or physical therapist. These measures may have to be employed throughout a lifetime to avoid or reduce pain. Obtain the advice of a tennis pro on proper equipment and technique.

Wear a tennis strap or band just below the elbow. The strap helps to constrict both the extensor and flexor muscles and takes the pressure off the areas at which these muscles attach to the elbow (lateral and medial epicondyles). This measure alone may greatly reduce pain.

Use an ice pack first to reduce swelling, then a heating pad to aid recovery.

See Your Physician: If pain is severe and limits forward motion of the arm.

SPORTS FIRST AID

FOOT

Morton's Neuroma (Pain in Forefoot)

What the Forefoot Is: The forefoot or front third of the foot is composed of five singular, long bones (metatarsals) that look like the fingers of your hand. The tips of these bones form the toes (phalanges).

What the Forefoot Does: The bones of the forefoot provide balance for the body.

Morton's Neuroma

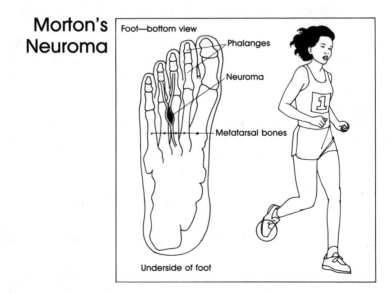

Foot—bottom view

Phalanges

Neuroma

Metatarsal bones

Underside of foot

Morton's neuroma is a swelling of a nerve between two metatarsal bones.

What the Condition Is: Morton's neuroma is a swelling of a nerve between two metatarsal bones.

Cause: Ill-fitting shoes and stress to the feet caused by repetitive athletic activity, as in running, are factors in Morton's neuroma. Genetic predisposition also can play a part: if the joints of the metatarsal bones are larger than usual, they may compress the nerve(s) between these bones—especially in athletic activity—and cause swelling of the nerve(s). The condition is common in many sports and not in one in particular. Other activities in which the condition can occur: wearing high heels—particularly shoes that crowd the toes—may make women more susceptible to this injury.

Symptoms: Pain on the top of the foot, in the ball of the foot, or in the toes. The pain may be severe and limit athletic participation. In some instances, the toes may become numb.

Immediate Treatment: *If pain is severe, if the toes are numb, or if walking produces severe pain, see your physician to determine proper treatment.*
   Stop the activity that is causing the pain. Remove your shoes. (Do not walk with shoes on.) Place an ice pack on the site of the pain as soon as possible. *Cold* treatments help stop internal bleeding and the accumulation of fluids in and around the injured area, thus decreasing swelling. Elevate the foot.

   Medication: (If you have seen your physician, follow his or her advice.) Take aspirin, ibuprofen, or acetaminophen to relieve pain and inflammation. Your physician may prescribe another mild analgesic (pain reliever) to help reduce pain or a nonsteroidal anti-inflammatory drug (NSAID) to help reduce pain and swelling. In some instances, your physician may suggest a low-dose injection of a corticosteroid or "steroid" drug, such as cortisone, that will help reduce inflammation.

NOTE: *Acetaminophen may not contain as much of the anti-inflammatory agents as aspirin or ibuprofen. Ask your physician or pharmacist for guidance.*

WARNING: *Do not give aspirin to children under the age of 16. If pregnant or nursing, consult with your physician first before taking medication.*

Continued Care: Rest the foot for 3 to 6 weeks. Use an ice pack on the injury at least once a day for 2 to 4 days after ceasing the activity, to reduce swelling and inflammation. Do not engage in original activity until pain has subsided. Use an ice pack to reduce any swelling that may occur.

Medication: Take aspirin, ibuprofen, or acetaminophen to relieve pain and inflammation.

Long-Term Effects of the Condition: None, with proper treatment and rest.

Prevention of Recurring Injury: The most important preventative measure is to wear shoes that give the foot room to move.

See Your Physician: If pain in foot or numbness in toes continues.

Plantar Fasciitis (Heel Spur)

What the Plantar Fascia Is: The plantar fascia is the long connective tissue on the bottom of the foot that extends from the calcaneus

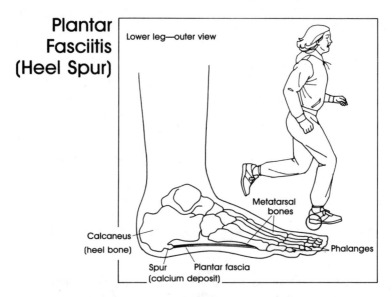

Plantar Fasciitis (Heel Spur)

Lower leg—outer view

Metatarsal bones

Calcaneus (heel bone)

Phalanges

Spur (calcium deposit)

Plantar fascia

Plantar fasciitis, or heel spur, is a tear in the plantar fascia that is aggravated by a spur that develops at the heel bone.

(heel bone), over the arch, to the ball of the foot and toes. The fascia forms part of the base of the foot.

What the Plantar Fascia Does: The fascia helps to support (and absorb shock to) the arch and foot during running, climbing, and jumping.

What the Injury Is: Plantar fasciitis, or heel spur, is a common ailment in sports. The injury can range from a microtear to a more serious—but rare—severing of the plantar fascia at the heel bone. Regardless of the extent of the tear, a spokelike calcium deposit, or "spur," can form at the heel bone, aggravating the condition.

Cause: The injury is usually caused by overuse, as in repetitive running. It also can be caused by poor arches, by wearing shoes with a stiff heel, or by running or competing in sports on unforgiving terrain (concrete, for example). It also can be caused by an increase in body weight. Other sports in which the injury can occur: aerobics, baseball, basketball, football, hiking, rugby, soccer, tennis, and track and field.

NOTE: *Women who regularly wear high heels and who do not stretch the calf muscles and the plantar fascia before engaging in sports may be prone to this injury.*

Symptoms: Pain at the heel, especially upon waking. Ironically, walking may hurt, but running, once the feet and legs have been warmed up, does not. Pain, however, may return the next morning. Bruises and swelling may be present on the heel. You may feel as if you are walking on a pea or a pebble.

Immediate Treatment: *If you are unable to place any pressure on the foot, or if walking or climbing stairs produces intense pain, see your physician to determine proper treatment.*

Stop the activity that is causing the pain. Place an ice pack on the heel as soon as possible. *Cold* treatments help stop internal bleeding and the accumulation of fluids in and around the injured area, thus decreasing swelling.

Medication: (If you have seen your physician, follow his or her advice.) Take aspirin, ibuprofen, or acetaminophen to relieve pain and inflammation. Your physician may prescribe another mild analgesic (pain reliever) to help reduce pain or a nonsteroidal anti-inflammatory drug (NSAID) to help reduce pain and swelling.

NOTE: *Acetaminophen may not contain as much of the anti-inflammatory agents as aspirin or ibuprofen. Ask your physician or pharmacist for guidance.*

WARNING: *Do not give aspirin to children under the age of 16. If pregnant or nursing, consult with your physician first before taking medication.*

Continued Care: Rest the foot for approximately 3 to 6 weeks. Use an ice pack at least once a day for 2 to 4 days after ceasing the activity, to reduce swelling and inflammation. Keep legs slightly elevated and extended straight out in front of you. (Keep off your feet as much as possible.) Do not engage in original activity until pain has subsided. With your physician's okay, work with a trainer or physical therapist on exercises that stretch the plantar fascia.

Medication: Take aspirin, ibuprofen, or acetaminophen to relieve pain and inflammation.

Long-Term Effects of Injury: Some pain and swelling may continue. In rare cases, surgery to release tension on the fascia, which involves severing the fascia from the heel bone, may be recommended.

Prevention of Recurring Injury: Allow plenty of time for the injury to heal. Your physician, trainer, or physical therapist may recommend shoe inserts to help relieve pressure on the heel while you are engaged in sports. Carefully perform exercises that stretch the calf muscles and the plantar fascia. Wear proper shoes. A stiff heel in running shoes or tennis shoes can cause or aggravate the condition. Run or train on a dirt track, not concrete.

See Your Physician: If pain and swelling continue.

Sprained Ankle

What the Ankle Is: The ankle consists of the fibula and tibia of the lower leg and the talus (anklebone) of the top of the foot. These bones form the ankle joint and are connected by a series of ligaments. Two important ligaments that help add stability to the joint are the anterior (outer) talofibular ligament, which runs from the outer ankle "knob" to the top of the foot, and the calcaneofibular ligament that connects the outer ankle knob to the calcaneus (heel bone).

What the Ankle Does: The ankle is a hinge joint that allows up-and-down flexion (bending) and limited side-to-side movement of the foot.

What the Injury Is: A sprained ankle is the most common injury in sports. The injury usually occurs to one or both ligaments located on the outside of the ankle and may range from a microtear to a complete severing of the ligaments from bone (with degrees of severity or tearing in between). A sprained ankle can be more painful than a break (or fracture) in a bone and may take as long to heal.

Cause: A sprain occurs when an athlete "rolls over" on the outside of the foot, causing the ligaments on the outside of the ankle to stretch or tear. The injury is common in all sports, including baseball, basketball, football, soccer, rugby, running, track and field, and tennis, and occurs in many activities outside of sports.

Symptoms: Pain, swelling, and bruising on the outside of the ankle and/or the top of the foot. At the onset of the sprain a hot flash may be felt on the outside of the ankle. Inability to walk. Ankle may feel warm for several hours. Depending upon the severity of the sprain, symptoms may appear immediately or 6 to 12 hours after the injury.

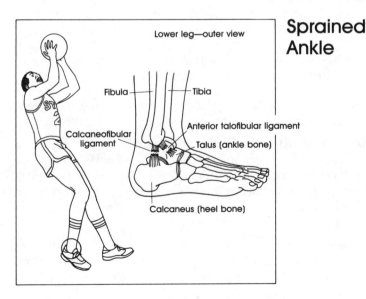

Lower leg—outer view

Sprained Ankle

Fibula

Tibia

Anterior talofibular ligament

Calcaneofibular ligament

Talus (ankle bone)

Calcaneus (heel bone)

SPORTS FIRST AID

A sprained ankle is an injury usually occurring to one or both ligaments located on the outside of the ankle.

Immediate Treatment: Stop the activity that has caused the sprain. Place an ice pack on the ankle as soon as possible after the injury. *Cold* treatments help stop internal bleeding and the accumulation of fluids in and around the injured area, thus decreasing swelling. See your physician to determine the severity of the sprain and to rule out a broken bone in the foot, ankle, or lower leg.

Medication: First, follow your physician's advice. Aspirin, ibuprofen, acetaminophen, another mild analgesic (pain reliever), or a nonsteroidal anti-inflammatory drug (NSAID) may be recommended to help reduce pain and swelling.

NOTE: *Acetaminophen may not contain as much of the anti-inflammatory agents as aspirin or ibuprofen. Ask your physician or pharmacist for guidance.*

WARNING: *Do not give aspirin to children under the age of 16. If pregnant or nursing, consult with your physician first before taking medication.*

Continued Care: Do not engage in the original activity until pain has subsided. Your physician may put a cast on the ankle to immobilize or restrict movement in the area. Or, your physician may recommend RICE (*r*est, *i*ce, *c*ompression, and *e*levation). Occasional use of an elastic bandage on the ankle may aid stability.

WARNING: *If you have vascular disease or diabetes, consult your physician first before using an elastic bandage.*

Medication: First, follow your physician's advice. Take aspirin, ibuprofen, or acetaminophen to relieve pain and inflammation.

Long-Term Effects of Injury: The ankle may be predisposed to recurrent sprains because of instability in the joint. (When the ligament stretches it usually does not return to its original shape.) It may also be predisposed to arthritis in the joint, caused by swelling and the development of bone "spurs" (small, spokelike calcium growths).

Prevention of Recurring Injury: Wear proper shoes (shoes that are not worn out). You may have to tape the ankle to aid stability. With your physician's okay, work with a trainer or physical therapist to strengthen the muscles around the ankle and lower calf.

See Your Physician: If pain and swelling continue.

Stress Fracture

What the Forefoot Is: The forefoot or front third of the foot is composed of five singular, long bones (metatarsals) that look like the fingers of your hand. The tips of these bones form the toes (phalanges).

What the Forefoot Does: The bones of the forefoot provide balance for the body.

What the Injury Is: A stress fracture usually occurs in the foot or in the tibia, one of the lower leg bones. A stress fracture in the foot is a hairline crack in one of the metatarsal bones.

Cause: A stress fracture in the foot can be caused by a repetitive motion over time, as in running, or by sudden stress placed on the foot, as in a change in running routine or surface, or as a result of participating in sports after a period of inactivity. It also can be caused by an increase in body weight. The condition is common in many sports other than running, including aerobics, baseball, basketball, tennis, rugby, soccer, and walking. Any activity that puts stress on the feet or legs over time may cause a stress fracture.

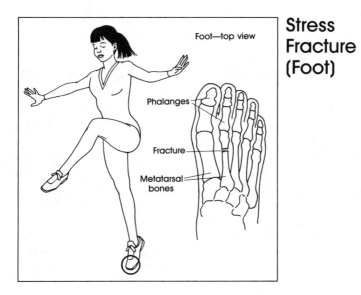

Foot—top view

Phalanges

Fracture

Metatarsal bones

Stress Fracture (Foot)

A stress fracture usually occurs in the foot or in the tibia, one of the lower leg bones. A stress fracture in the foot is a hairline crack in one of the metatarsal bones.

Symptoms: Intense pain at the point of the fracture. During exercise, the foot or leg may feel as if it is on fire. Pain may subside when you stop the activity. In more serious cases, the pain may continue even though you have ceased the activity.

Immediate Treatment: *If pain is severe and inhibits walking, see your physician to determine proper treatment.* Stop the activity that is causing the pain. Place an ice pack on the site of the pain as soon as possible. *Cold* treatments help stop internal bleeding and the accumulation of fluids in and around the injured area, thus decreasing swelling.

Medication: (If you have seen your physician, follow his or her advice.) Take aspirin, ibuprofen, or acetaminophen to relieve pain and inflammation. Your physician may prescribe another mild analgesic (pain reliever) to help reduce pain or a nonsteroidal anti-inflammatory drug (NSAID) to help reduce pain and swelling.

NOTE: *Acetaminophen may not contain as much of the anti-inflammatory agents as aspirin or ibuprofen. Ask your physician or pharmacist for guidance.*

WARNING: *Do not give aspirin to children under the age of 16. If pregnant or nursing, consult with your physician first before taking medication.*

Continued Care: Rest the foot for 4 to 6 weeks. Use an ice pack at the site of the pain at least once a day to help reduce pain and inflammation. Do not engage in original activity until pain has subsided. Use an ice pack to reduce any swelling that may occur.

Medication: Take aspirin, ibuprofen, or acetaminophen to relieve pain and inflammation.

Long-Term Effects of Injury: None, with proper treatment and rest.

Prevention of Recurring Injury: Resume activity gradually, especially the running sports. Wear proper shoes. Run or train on a forgiving surface, such as a dirt track. Increase any speed or distance (as in running) gradually.

See Your Physician: If pain continues after you resume activity.

HAND

Baseball Finger (Mallet Finger)

What the Hand Is: The hand consists of the bones and joints of the fingers and thumb (called phalanges), the five metacarpal bones of the palm, and eight small, oblong-shaped bones that, together, form the wrist. Beneath the skin is a complex network of ligaments, tendons, and muscles.

What the Hand Does: Empowered from the muscles in the forearm, the hand allows a wide range of motion and tasks.

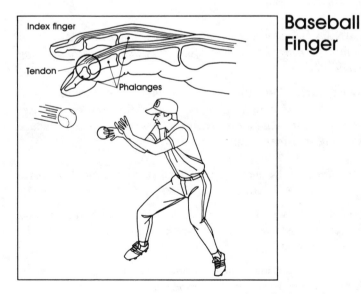

Baseball Finger

Baseball finger, in which a tendon rips away from the bone, is caused by a blow to the end of the finger.

What the Injury Is: Baseball finger is a tear in a tendon at the joint at the end of the finger. Depending upon the severity of the injury, you may not be able to straighten the finger.

Cause: The injury is caused by sudden force exerted on the end of the finger, such as from a thrown or hit baseball.

Symptoms: Immediate pain at the site of the injury. Swelling. Bruising.

Immediate Treatment: Place an ice pack on the finger as soon as possible after the injury. *Cold* treatments help stop internal bleeding and the accumulation of fluids in and around the injured area, thus decreasing swelling. See your physician to determine the extent of the injury. Your physician may advise the use of a splint on the finger to aid healing.

Medication: (If you have seen your physician, follow his or her advice.) Take aspirin, ibuprofen, or acetaminophen regularly to relieve pain and inflammation.

NOTE: *Acetaminophen may not contain as much of the anti-inflammatory agents as aspirin or ibuprofen. Ask your physician or pharmacist for guidance.*

WARNING: *Do not give aspirin to children under the age of 16. If pregnant or nursing, consult with your physician first before taking any medication.*

Continued Care: Do not engage in the original activity until pain has subsided. Work with a trainer or physical therapist on exercises that strengthen the tendons in the fingers. Use an ice pack to reduce any swelling that may occur.

Medication: Take aspirin, ibuprofen, or acetaminophen to relieve pain and inflammation.

Long-Term Effects of Injury: None, with proper treatment and rest. In serious cases, surgery may be recommended to reattach the tendon to the bone.

Prevention of Recurring Injury: Continue exercises that strengthen the tendons in the finger. Use good judgment in your sport.

See Your Physician: If pain continues or reinjury occurs.

Skier's Thumb (Gamekeeper's Thumb)

What the Hand Is: The hand consists of the bones and joints of the fingers and thumb (called phalanges), the five metacarpal bones of the palm, and eight small, oblong-shaped bones that, together, form the wrist. Beneath the skin is a complex network of ligaments, tendons, and muscles.

What the Hand Does: Empowered from the muscles in the forearm, the hand allows a wide range of motion and tasks.

What the Injury Is: Skier's thumb is a tear in the ligament—or, more seriously, a complete severing of the ligament—that attaches the thumb to one of the metacarpal bones.

Cause: The injury is commonly caused in skiing during a fall, in which the ski pole forces the thumb away from the fingers. It can also occur when catching a swiftly thrown baseball, football, or basketball. (A century ago in Europe, gamekeepers—using the thumb and index finger—broke the necks of small animals caught in traps and suffered the same malady.)

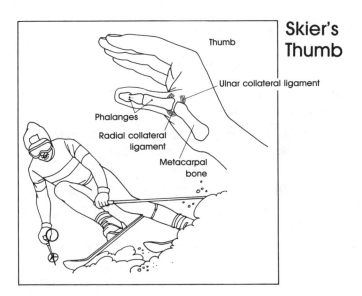

Thumb

Skier's Thumb

Ulnar collateral ligament

Phalanges

Radial collateral ligament

Metacarpal bone

Skier's thumb is a tear in the ligament—or, more seriously, a complete severing of the ligament—that attaches the thumb to the metacarpal bone.

SPORTS FIRST AID

Symptoms: Immediate pain at the base of the thumb. Swelling. Pain may intensify and bruising may occur several hours after the injury.

Immediate Treatment: Place an ice pack on the base of the thumb as soon as possible after the injury. *Cold* treatments help stop internal bleeding and the accumulation of fluids in and around the injured area, thus decreasing swelling. See your physician to determine the extent of the injury. Your physician may advise the use of a splint on the thumb to aid healing.

Medication: (If you have seen your physician, follow his or her advice.) Take aspirin, ibuprofen, or acetaminophen regularly to relieve pain and inflammation.

NOTE: *Acetaminophen may not contain as much of the anti-inflammatory agents as aspirin or ibuprofen. Ask your physician or pharmacist for guidance.*

WARNING: *Do not give aspirin to children under the age of 16. If pregnant or nursing, consult with your physician first before taking any medication.*

Continued Care: Do not engage in the original activity until pain has subsided. Work with a trainer or physical therapist on exercises that strengthen the tendons and ligaments in the hand. Use an ice pack to reduce any swelling that may occur.

Medication: Take aspirin, ibuprofen, or acetaminophen to relieve pain and inflammation.

Long-Term Effects of Injury: None, with proper treatment and rest. In serious cases, surgery will be necessary to repair the ligament.

Prevention of Recurring Injury: Continue exercises that strengthen the tendons and ligaments in the hand. Use good judgment in your sport.

See Your Physician: If pain continues or reinjury occurs.

HIP

Hip Pointer

What the Hip Is: The hip consists of the ilium bone (the top of the pelvis), the sacrum and coccyx (tailbone) of the lower spine, the pubic bone, and the ischium bone (the bottom of the pelvis). Connected to the hip are several muscle-tendon groups.

What the Hip Does: The bones of the hip protect the internal organs of the body and allow us to stand and move.

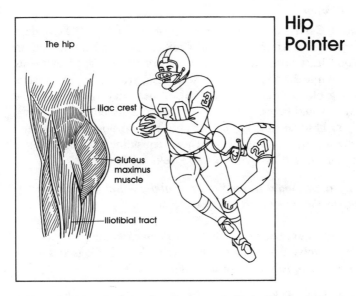

Hip Pointer

The hip

Iliac crest

Gluteus maximus muscle

Iliotibial tract

A hip pointer is a bruise or tear in a muscle that attaches to the top of the ilium bone, at the waist.

What the Injury Is: A hip pointer is a bruise or tear in a muscle that attaches to the top of the ilium bone, at the waist.

Cause: The injury, very common in contact sports, is caused by a blow to or a fall on the hip.

Symptoms: Pain at the hip. Pain may intensify several hours after the injury. Bruising at the hip.

Immediate Treatment: *If pain is severe and inhibits walking, see your physician to determine proper treatment.* Place an ice pack on the hipbone as soon as possible after the injury. *Cold* treatments help stop internal bleeding and the accumulation of fluids in and around the injured area, thus decreasing swelling.

Medication: (If you have seen your physician, follow his or her advice.) Take aspirin, ibuprofen, or acetaminophen regularly to relieve pain and inflammation.

NOTE: *Acetaminophen may not contain as much of the anti-inflammatory agents as aspirin or ibuprofen. Ask your physician or pharmacist for guidance.*

WARNING: *Do not give aspirin to children under the age of 16. If pregnant or nursing, consult with your physician first before taking any medication.*

Continued Care: Use an ice pack at least once a day for 2 to 4 days after the injury. After swelling has ceased, place a heating pad on the hip at least once a day until the injury heals. *Heat* treatments help to enlarge the small blood vessels in and around the injury, thus increasing blood circulation. (Blood carries vital nutrients to the injured area and helps speed recovery.) Avoid athletic activity until the injury has had time to heal, or until there is no pain in the hip. The length of time for the injury to heal, depending upon the severity of the tear, may range from 3 to 6 weeks, or longer.

NOTE: *Heat should be applied only after swelling has subsided or swelling in the injured area may increase.*

After the injury has healed, gradually and carefully perform exercises that involve stretching the muscles in the upper legs and waist. Use an ice pack to reduce any swelling.

Medication: Take aspirin, ibuprofen, or acetaminophen to relieve pain and inflammation.

Long-Term Effects of Injury: None, with proper rest.

Prevention of Recurring Injury: Wear hip padding if you are engaging in contact sports. Avoid falls on the hip.

See Your Physician: If pain continues or if reinjury occurs.

SPORTS FIRST AID

KNEE

Runner's Knee

What the Knee Is: The knee consists of three main bones, the femur of the upper leg and the tibia and fibula of the lower leg. These bones are connected by a series of ligaments—connective tissue—to form the knee joint. Resting on top of this joint is a fourth bone, the patella (kneecap). Bursas—fluid-filled sacs or saclike cavities—sur-

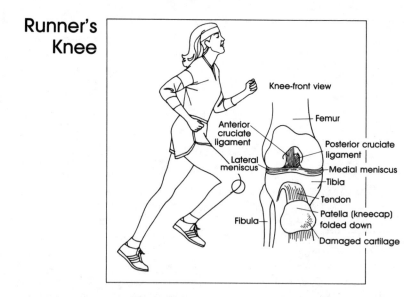

Runner's Knee

Knee-front view

Femur

Anterior cruciate ligament

Posterior cruciate ligament

Lateral meniscus

Medial meniscus

Tibia

Tendon

Fibula

Patella (kneecap) folded down

Damaged cartilage

Runner's knee—pain on or behind the knee—is caused by damage to cartilage that covers the under surface of the kneecap. It can also be pain on the outside of one or both knees.

round and cushion the bones. Muscles, such as the quadriceps in the front upper leg and the hamstrings in the back upper leg, are connected to these bones by tendons (also connective tissue). The muscles, tendons, and ligaments all add stability to the joint.

What the Knee Does: The knee, like the elbow, is a hinge joint that allows extension and flexion (bending) of the leg.

What the Condition Is: Runner's knee, or chondromalacia, is a common ailment that afflicts runners and other athletes of all abilities. The term refers to damage to and roughness of the cartilage that covers the under surface of the kneecap. (Cartilage covers all bone and joint surfaces and acts as a shock absorber to keep bone from rubbing against bone.) When this condition occurs, rough spots on the kneecap can rub directly against the femur, causing pain.*

Cause: The condition can be caused by either a repetitive motion over time, as in running, or sudden stress placed on the knee, as in a change in running routine or surface, using heavier weights in weight lifting, or using a high gear in bicycling. It also may be caused by genetic factors (loose kneecap or an abnormality in the structure of the kneecap), by a direct or forceful blow to the kneecap, or as a result of unknown factors.

Other sports that can cause runner's knee: any sport in which pressure is put on the knees, as in weight lifting, football, tennis, rowing, aerobics, or bicycling. Other activities that may cause runner's knee: heavy lifting or stair climbing over time.

Symptoms: Anything from a dull ache to a sharp pain on and behind the kneecap. Pain while sitting with the knees bent. Pain when kneeling or squatting. Pain when walking upstairs or downstairs. Swelling on the knee. Muscle weakness in the quadriceps. Grinding and popping of the knee.

---

*Runner's knee has also been described as pain on the outside of one or both knees. This condition, though not as common as chondromalacia, is usually caused by "overuse"—increasing running mileage, for example, without acclimating first to the new distance. It occurs when the foot strikes the ground at a pronounced angle while running, causing pain at the knee. (Usually, the outside of the shoe and the heel are worn down.) This results in stress to and a possible microtear in the iliotibial band—a connective tissue that extends from the ilium (hip bone) to the top of the tibia.

The condition can be corrected with shoe inserts—molding that fits inside the shoe that gives your foot support and helps you strike the ground properly while running. See your physician, however, for proper diagnosis and treatment.

SPORTS FIRST AID

Immediate Treatment: *If pain is persistent, severe, and makes walking upstairs or downstairs very difficult, see your physician to determine proper treatment.* RICE—rest, ice, compression, and elevation. Stop the activity that is causing the pain. Place an ice pack on the knee as soon as possible. *Cold* treatments help stop internal bleeding and the accumulation of fluids in and around the injured area, thus decreasing swelling.

Medication: (If you have seen your physician, follow his or her advice.) Take aspirin, ibuprofen, or acetaminophen to relieve pain and inflammation. Your physician may prescribe another mild analgesic (pain reliever) to help reduce pain or a nonsteroidal anti-inflammatory drug (NSAID) to help reduce pain and swelling.

NOTE: *Acetaminophen may not contain as much of the anti-inflammatory agents as aspirin or ibuprofen. Ask your physician or pharmacist for guidance.*

WARNING: *Do not give aspirin to children under the age of 16. If pregnant or nursing, consult with your physician first before taking any medication.*

Continued Care: Rest the legs for approximately 3 to 6 weeks. Use ice for 2 to 4 days after ceasing the activity to reduce swelling and inflammation. Occasional use of an elastic bandage on the knee may help add stability. Keep legs slightly elevated.

WARNING: *If you have vascular disease or diabetes, consult your physician first before using an elastic bandage.*

Do not engage in the original activity until pain has subsided. With your physician's okay, work with a trainer or physical therapist on exercises that strengthen the quadriceps muscles. Use an ice pack to reduce any swelling that may occur.

Medication: Take aspirin, ibuprofen, or acetaminophen to relieve pain and inflammation.

Long-Term Effects of the Condition: Some pain may continue when the knee is bent. You may have difficulty kneeling or squatting. In some cases surgery may be recommended to smooth the roughness on the back of the kneecap. (Cartilage does not heal on its own.)

Prevention of Recurring Injury: Use good judgment in increasing running mileage and intensity or in changing to a different surface or terrain. Don't "push the high gears" in bicycling. Gradually acclimate to lifting heavy objects. Ensure that shoes fit properly. Keep quadriceps muscles strong. Muscle-strengthening exercises also help strengthen ligaments and tendons.

See Your Physician: If pain and swelling continue.

Torn Cartilage

What the Knee Is: The knee consists of three main bones, the femur of the upper leg and the tibia and fibula of the lower leg. These bones are connected by a series of ligaments—connective tissue—to form the knee joint. Resting on top of this joint is a fourth bone, the patella (kneecap). Bursas—fluid-filled sacs or saclike cavities—surround and cushion the bones. Muscles, such as the quadriceps in the front upper leg and the hamstrings in the back upper leg, are connected to these bones by tendons (also connective tissue). The muscles, tendons, and ligaments all add stability to the joint.

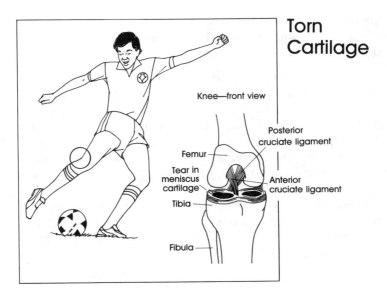

Torn Cartilage

Knee—front view

Posterior cruciate ligament
Femur
Tear in meniscus cartilage
Anterior cruciate ligament
Tibia
Fibula

A torn cartilage in the knee is usually caused by a severe twist or forceful blow to the knee when the leg is hyperextended (straightened).

SPORTS FIRST AID

What the Knee Does: The knee, like the elbow, is a hinge joint that allows extension and flexion (bending) of the leg.

What the Injury Is: The injury occurs in the meniscus cartilage—a circular band of elastic material that sits on top of the tibia. This cartilage helps the knee joint fit snugly together and helps distribute body weight evenly over the surface of the tibia. The injury can range from a microtear to a complete tear in the cartilage, the latter, in most cases, requiring surgery to repair. (Cartilage does not heal on its own.) What may begin as a small tear can, with repeated twists or blows to the knee, develop into a complete tear.

Cause: The injury is usually caused by a severe twist or forceful blow to the knee when the leg is hyperextended (straightened). It also can occur from force placed on the knee by the athlete himself or herself when the foot is planted, the leg straightened, and the knee then twisted, as in downhill skiing or playing basketball. Torn cartilage sometimes occurs in conjunction with a torn ligament in the knee. The injury is very common in contact sports and among athletes of all abilities. Other sports in which the injury can occur: football, hockey, lacrosse, soccer, and golf. Other situations in which the injury can occur: tripping over objects on the floor or ground; falling with force on the knee.

Symptoms: Pain at the joint line (the area at which the bones of the leg join to form the knee). The knee may lock or buckle. The athlete may hear a popping sound. Swelling may occur.

Immediate Treatment: Stop the activity that is causing the pain. (In most instances, pain and swelling will prohibit you from continuing.) Apply an ice pack to the knee. (*Cold* treatments help stop internal bleeding and the accumulation of fluids in and around the injured area, thus decreasing swelling.) See a physician for proper diagnosis of the extent of the tear. Surgery may be recommended to repair or remove the damaged cartilage.

Medication: First, follow your physician's advice. Aspirin, ibuprofen, acetaminophen, another mild analgesic (pain reliever), or a nonsteroidal anti-inflammatory drug (NSAID) may be recommended to help reduce pain and swelling.

NOTE: *Acetaminophen may not contain as much of the anti-inflammatory agents as aspirin or ibuprofen. Ask your physician or pharmacist for guidance.*

WARNING: *Do not give aspirin to children under the age of 16. If pregnant or nursing, consult with your physician first before taking any medication.*

Continued Care: Follow your physician's instructions regarding care.

Medication: First, follow your physician's advice. Take aspirin, ibuprofen, or acetaminophen to relieve pain and inflammation.

Long-Term Effects of Injury: Some stiffness and swelling may recur. The injury may predispose you to arthritis and to ligament tears in the knee.

Prevention of Recurring Injury: With your physician's okay, work with a trainer or physical therapist to strengthen the hamstring muscles on the back upper leg and the quadriceps muscles on the front upper leg.

See Your Physician: If pain and swelling continue after the injury. If the knee locks or buckles.

Torn Ligament

What the Knee Is: The knee consists of three main bones, the femur of the upper leg and the tibia and fibula of the lower leg. These bones are connected by a series of ligaments—connective tissue—to form the knee joint. Resting on top of this joint is a fourth bone, the patella (kneecap). Bursas—fluid-filled sacs or saclike cavities—surround and cushion the bones. Muscles, such as the quadriceps in the front upper leg and the hamstrings in the back upper leg, are connected to these bones by tendons (also connective tissue). The muscles, tendons, and ligaments all add stability to the joint.

What the Knee Does: The knee, like the elbow, is a hinge joint that allows extension and flexion (bending) of the leg.

What the Injury Is: Damage to the anterior cruciate ligament—also referred to as an ACL injury—is one of the most common injuries in sports next to a sprained ankle. This ligament is one of two ligaments that crisscross behind the knee and add stability to the knee joint. Damage may range from a microtear to a full severing of the ligament from the bone (with degrees of severity or tearing

SPORTS FIRST AID

in between). A tear in the ligament may also be accompanied by torn cartilage in the knee.

Cause: The injury is caused by a traumatic or sudden blow to the knee when the leg is hyperextended (straightened). It also can occur from force placed on the knee by the athlete himself or herself when the foot is planted and the leg is straightened, as in downhill skiing or playing basketball.

   The injury is very common in contact sports and among athletes of all abilities. Other sports in which the injury can occur: football, lacrosse, soccer. Other situations in which the injury can occur: tripping over the cat or dog.

Symptoms: Swelling and pain from the accumulation of fluid and blood inside the knee. Limitation of motion. Stiffness. May hear or feel a popping sound when the ligament is torn. Knee may go out of place. Depending upon the severity of the tear, symptoms may not appear for 6 to 12 hours.

Immediate Treatment: Stop the activity that is causing the pain. Apply an ice pack to the knee. *Cold* treatments help stop internal

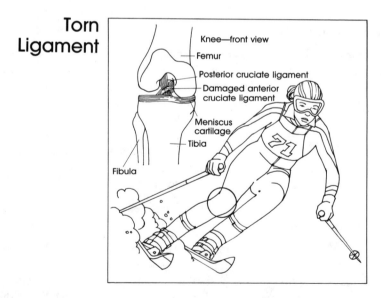

Torn Ligament

Knee—front view
Femur
Posterior cruciate ligament
Damaged anterior cruciate ligament
Meniscus cartilage
Tibia
Fibula

Damage to the anterior cruciate ligament—also referred to as an ACL injury—is a common occurrence in sports. The ligament adds stability to the knee joint.

bleeding and the accumulation of fluids in and around the injured area, thus decreasing swelling. See a physician for proper diagnosis of the extent of the tear. Surgery may be recommended to repair the ligament.

Medication: First, follow your physician's advice. Aspirin, ibuprofen, acetaminophen, another mild analgesic (pain reliever), or a nonsteroidal anti-inflammatory drug (NSAID) may be recommended to help reduce pain and swelling.

NOTE: *Acetaminophen may not contain as much of the anti-inflammatory agents as aspirin or ibuprofen. Ask your physician or pharmacist for guidance.*

WARNING: *Do not give aspirin to children under the age of 16. If pregnant or nursing, consult with your physician first before taking any medication.*

Continued Care: Follow your physician's instructions regarding care.

Medication: First, follow your physician's advice. Take aspirin, ibuprofen, or acetaminophen to relieve pain and inflammation.

Long-Term Effects of Injury: The knee may be unstable. It may "give out," especially when you are engaged in a sharp turn to the left or right, as in "cutting" in football. You may be predisposed to cartilage tears because the knee is loose.

Prevention of Recurring Injury: With your physician's okay, work with a trainer or physical therapist to strengthen the leg muscles, especially the hamstring muscles on the back upper leg. Muscle-strengthening exercises also help strengthen ligaments and tendons.

See Your Physician: If pain and swelling continue in the knee after the injury. If the knee buckles. If you suspect that you have torn the ligament.

SPORTS FIRST AID

LEG

Achilles Tendinitis

What the Achilles Tendon Is: The achilles tendon attaches the gastrocnemius, plantar, and soleus muscles—the calf muscles—of the lower part of the leg to the calcaneus (heel bone). The Achilles tendon is one of the longest tendons in the body.

What the Achilles Tendon Does: The tendon allows you to run, climb, and stand on the tips of your toes.

Achilles Tendinitis

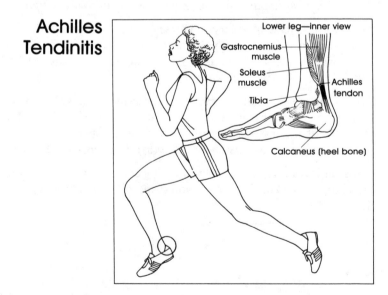

Lower leg—inner view

Gastrocnemius muscle

Soleus muscle

Tibia

Achilles tendon

Calcaneus (heel bone)

Achilles tendinitis is a strain or tear in the tendon that attaches the calf muscles to the heel bone.

What the Injury Is: Injury to the Achilles tendon can range from a microtear to a more serious—but rare—severing of the tendon from the heel bone (with degrees of strain or tearing in between).

Cause: The injury can be caused by a repetitive motion over time, as in running, or by sudden stress placed on the tendon, as in sprinting. A tear can also occur if the tendon is fatigued from overuse; if pressure is placed upon it without a sufficient warm-up period; from wearing improper shoes during sports; from wearing athletic shoes with a stiff heel; or from running or training on a hard surface. The injury can occur in any sport, but particularly in aerobics, baseball, basketball, football, hiking, rugby, soccer, tennis, and track and field. Other activities can also cause the injury, such as running for the bus, or taking long walks without acclimating first to the distance.

Symptoms: Symptoms range from mild discomfort to severe pain depending upon the extent of the tear. Pain may be centered at the lower back of the leg above the ankle. With a mild strain or tear, pain may be noticeable upon waking, but as the tendon warms up during walking or exercise, the pain may disappear. Discomfort, however, may return the next morning. With a more serious tear or severing of the tendon, you may feel as if someone kicked you in the back of the leg as the tendon ruptures. With both minor and major injuries to the tendon, pain and swelling—from the accumulation of fluids—will worsen several hours after the onset of the injury.

Immediate Treatment: *If pain is severe or if you are unable to walk or climb stairs, see your physician to determine proper treatment.* Stop the activity that is causing the pain. Place an ice pack on the site of the injury as soon as possible. *Cold* treatments help stop internal bleeding and the accumulation of fluids in and around the injured area, thus decreasing swelling.

Medication: (If you have seen your physician, follow his or her advice.) Take aspirin, ibuprofen, or acetaminophen regularly to relieve pain and inflammation. Your physician may prescribe another mild analgesic (pain reliever) to help reduce pain or a nonsteroidal anti-inflammatory drug (NSAID) to help reduce pain and swelling.

NOTE: *Acetaminophen may not contain as much of the anti-inflammatory agents as aspirin or ibuprofen. Ask your physician or pharmacist for guidance.*

SPORTS FIRST AID

WARNING: *Do not give aspirin to children under the age of 16. If pregnant or nursing, consult with your physician first before taking medication.*

Continued Care: Place an ice pack on the site of the injury at least once a day for 2 to 4 days after ceasing the activity, to reduce swelling and inflammation. Do not engage in original activity until pain has subsided. Gradually and carefully extend or stretch your lower leg and foot. Work with a trainer or physical therapist on light exercises that stretch the calf muscles and the Achilles tendon. Use an ice pack to reduce any swelling that may occur.

Medication: Take aspirin, ibuprofen, or acetaminophen to relieve pain and inflammation.

Long-Term Effects of Injury: None, with proper treatment and rest, although some individuals may suffer recurring tendinitis regardless of precautionary measures. In rare cases, surgery may be recommended to remove scar tissue and part of the tendon.

Prevention of Recurring Injury: Allow plenty of time for the injury to heal. Your physician, trainer, or physical therapist may recommend shoe inserts to help relieve pressure on the heel while you are engaged in sports. Carefully perform exercises that stretch the calf muscles and the Achilles tendon. Wear proper shoes. A stiff heel in running shoes or tennis shoes can cause or aggravate the condition. Run or train on a dirt track, not concrete.

See Your Physician: If pain and swelling continue.

Hamstring Muscle Pull

What the Hamstring Is: The hamstring is the large muscle on the back of the thigh that runs from the bottom of the pelvis to the top of the knee. About mid-thigh, the muscle separates into two major muscle-tendon groups. The medial (inner) hamstring tendons attach to the inner knee and the front of the tibia (one of the lower leg bones). The other, the lateral (outer) hamstring tendons, attach to the outside of the knee at the top of the fibula (the other lower leg bone).

What the Hamstring Does: The hamstring muscle flexes (bends) the leg. (The quadriceps muscle on the front of the thigh expands or straightens the leg.)

What the Injury Is: Injury to the hamstring can range from a microtear to a more serious tear in the muscle or in the tendons that attach the muscle to bone. Most injuries to the hamstring, however, occur in the muscle.

Cause: The injury is common among athletes of all abilities. It usually occurs from a quick start when the leg is hyperextended (straightened), as in sprinting, rather than from a repetitive motion over time, as in running. The injury can be caused when the quadriceps muscle is overdeveloped in relation to the hamstring muscle or from engaging in sports without a sufficient warm-up period. Some individuals have naturally tight hamstrings that *may or may not* make them more susceptible to injury. Other sports in which a hamstring injury can occur: baseball, football, basketball, rugby, soccer, and tennis.

Symptoms. Pain in the back of the leg. The degree of pain will depend upon the severity of the tear. With some tears or strains in the muscle, pain may worsen over several hours. It may be difficult to walk, sit, or bend over.

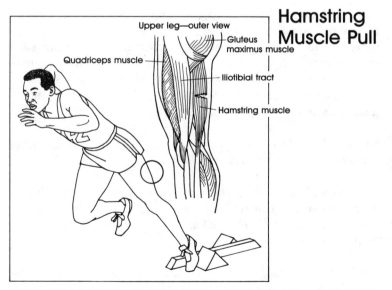

Upper leg—outer view

Gluteus maximus muscle

Quadriceps muscle

Iliotibial tract

Hamstring muscle

Hamstring
Muscle Pull

Injury to the hamstring can range from a microtear to a more serious tear in the muscle or in the tendons that attach the muscle to bone.

Immediate Treatment: *If pain is severe in the back of the leg or if you cannot straighten your leg to walk, see your physician to determine proper treatment.* RICE (rest, ice, compression, and elevation). Stop the activity that is causing the pain. Place an ice pack on the back of the leg as soon as possible.

Cold treatments help stop internal bleeding and the accumulation of fluids in and around the injured area, thus decreasing swelling.

Medication: (If you have seen your physician, follow his or her advice.) Take aspirin, ibuprofen, or acetaminophen regularly to relieve pain and inflammation.

Your physician may prescribe another mild analgesic (pain reliever) to help reduce pain or a nonsteroidal anti-inflammatory drug (NSAID) to help reduce pain and swelling.

NOTE: *Acetaminophen may not contain as much of the anti-inflammatory agents as aspirin or ibuprofen. Ask your physician or pharmacist for guidance.*

WARNING: *Do not give aspirin to children under the age of 16. If pregnant or nursing, consult with your physician first before taking medication.*

Continued Care: Rest the legs for approximately 1 to 3 weeks, depending upon the extent of the injury. Use an ice pack at least once a day for 2 to 4 days after ceasing the activity to reduce swelling and inflammation. Use a heating pad thereafter. *Heat* treatments help to enlarge the small blood vessels in and around the injury, thus increasing blood circulation. (Blood carries vital nutrients to the injured area and helps speed recovery.)

NOTE: *Heat should be applied only after swelling has subsided, or swelling in the injured area may increase.*

Occasional use of an elastic bandage on the upper leg will help relieve pressure by compressing the quadriceps and hamstring muscles. Keep legs slightly elevated and extended straight out in front of you when you can.

WARNING: *If you have vascular disease or diabetes, consult your physician first before using an elastic bandage. (An elastic bandage can constrict blood circulation.)*

Do not engage in original activity until pain has subsided. Gradually and carefully bend and stretch your leg. Work with a trainer or physical therapist on light exercises that strengthen the hamstring and quadriceps muscles. Use an ice pack to reduce any swelling that may occur.

Medication: Take aspirin, ibuprofen, or acetaminophen to relieve pain and inflammation.

Long-Term Effects of Injury: None, with proper rest and rehabilitation.

Prevention of Recurring Injury: Warm up properly. Perform exercises that strengthen the hamstring and quadriceps muscles.

See Your Physician: If pain continues or reinjury occurs.

Shin Splint

What the Shin Is: The shin is the front portion of the leg below the knee. It consists primarily of the two large bones of the lower leg, the fibula and tibia.

What the Shin Does: The bones of the lower leg provide support for the body and, through ligaments and muscles, serve as the attachment point for the foot.

What the Injury Is: While not a medical term, "shin splint" denotes the anatomical location of pain that occurs in the front of the lower leg. A shin splint can be one of several injuries: a microtear in a muscle (the posterior tibial muscle) at the point at which it attaches to the tibia on the front of the leg; a stress fracture in the bone; a microtear or inflammation in the thin membrane (periosteum) that covers all of the body's bone surfaces; or an anterior compartment syndrome, in which the muscles, during exercise, become too large for the area in which they reside. In serious cases of compartment syndrome, blood flow to and from the muscles can be restricted.

Cause: A tear in the muscle, a stress fracture in the bone, or a microtear or inflammation in the membrane covering the bone can all be caused by overuse, such as running repetitively without rest; by a change in running routine or surface; or by participating in sports after a period of inactivity. The injury can also be caused by an increase in body weight. Compartment syndrome is caused when exercise increases the size of the muscle mass in the lower leg, causing the muscles to strain against bone and fascia (a membrane that covers all of the body's muscles). Shin splints are common among athletes of all abilities and occur in many sports other than running, including aerobics, baseball, basketball, tennis, rugby, soccer, and walking.

Symptoms: Pain in the lower front portion of the leg.

Immediate Treatment: *If pain in the leg is severe or if you are unable to walk, see your physician to rule out a stress fracture or anterior compartment syndrome.* Stop the activity that is causing the pain. Use an ice pack at the site of the injury to help reduce pain and inflammation. *Cold* treatments help stop internal bleeding and the accumulation of fluids in and around the injured area, thus decreasing swelling.

Medication: (If you have seen your physician, follow his or her advice.) Take aspirin, ibuprofen, or acetaminophen to relieve pain and inflammation. Your physician may prescribe another mild anal-

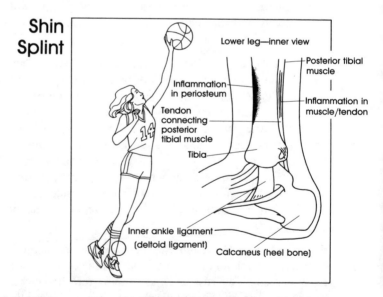

Shin
Splint

Lower leg—inner view

Posterior tibial muscle

Inflammation in periosteum

Inflammation in muscle/tendon

Tendon connecting posterior tibial muscle

Tibia

Inner ankle ligament (deltoid ligament)

Calcaneus (heel bone)

A shin splint can be one of several injuries: a microtear in a muscle, a stress fracture in the lower leg bone, a microtear or an inflammation in the membrane that covers the bone surface, or overdevelopment of the leg muscle.

gesic (pain reliever) to help reduce pain or a nonsteroidal anti-inflammatory drug (NSAID) to help reduce pain and swelling.

NOTE: *Acetaminophen may not contain as much of the anti-inflammatory agents as aspirin or ibuprofen. Ask your physician or pharmacist for guidance.*

WARNING: *Do not give aspirin to children under the age of 16. If pregnant or nursing, consult with your physician first before taking medication.*

Continued Care: Rest the legs for 3 to 6 weeks. Use an ice pack at least once a day for 2 to 4 days after the injury. Use a heating pad thereafter. *Heat* treatments help to enlarge the small blood vessels in and around the injury, thus increasing blood circulation. (Blood carries vital nutrients to the injured area and helps speed recovery.)

NOTE: *Heat should be applied only after the swelling has subsided, or swelling in the injured area may increase.*

Do not engage in original activity until pain has subsided. Use an ice pack to reduce any swelling that may occur.

Medication: Take aspirin, ibuprofen, or acetaminophen to relieve pain and inflammation.

Long-Term Effects of Injury: None, with proper treatment and rest. In serious cases of anterior compartment syndrome, surgery may be required to cut the fascia covering the muscle.

Prevention of Recurring Injury: Work with a trainer or physical therapist to strengthen the surrounding ankle muscles. You may be advised to use shoe inserts that will help support the arch and take stress off the lower leg. Resume any activity gradually, especially the running sports.

See Your Physician: If pain continues after you resume activity.

SPORTS FIRST AID

MUSCLES

Muscle Cramps

Where Muscle Cramps Occur: Muscle cramps can occur almost anywhere in the body. During athletic activity, cramps can occur in the stomach, legs, feet, arms, neck, or back. Cramps in the legs are very common, particularly in the hamstring muscles in the back, upper leg; the quadriceps muscles in the front, upper leg; and the calf muscles in the back of the lower leg.

Muscle Cramps

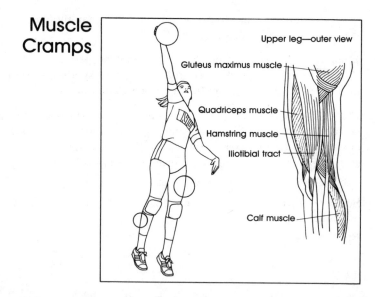

Upper leg—outer view

Gluteus maximus muscle

Quadriceps muscle

Hamstring muscle

Iliotibial tract

Calf muscle

Muscle cramps occur when the muscles tighten up during (or because of) continuous athletic activity.

What Muscles Do: Muscles and muscle-tendon groups provide the means for the body to move.

What a Muscle Cramp Is: Muscle cramps occur when the muscles tighten up during (or because of) continuous athletic activity. Cramps occur when the muscles deplete their store of oxygen and glycogen—a carbohydrate energy source stored in muscles and in the liver. Cramps can also occur with an electrolyte (body chemical) imbalance, or when the body has insufficient water to help remove waste products.

Cause: Cramps occur most often from overuse—during a marathon road race, an extended tennis match, or a long bicycle ride, for example.

Symptoms: Muscle cramps can be very painful. If the activity that is causing the cramp is stopped, the cramp can become worse. However, continuation of the activity is often impossible.

Immediate Treatment: *Some cramping can be severe. If the cramp is not relieved by massage, or if a heating pad is not available to place on the muscle, take the individual to the nearest hospital emergency room for treatment.* Gently stretch out the muscle if possible. Massage the muscle to help work out the cramp. If a heating pad is available, place it on the cramped muscle to help relieve tightness. Continue massaging the muscle until the cramp goes away.

Medication: (If you have seen your physician, follow his or her advice.) Take aspirin, ibuprofen, or acetaminophen to help relieve pain and inflammation.

NOTE: *Acetaminophen may not contain as much of the anti-inflammatory agents as aspirin or ibuprofen. Ask your physician or pharmacist for guidance.*

WARNING: *Do not give aspirin to children under the age of 16. If pregnant or nursing, consult with your physician first before taking any medication.*

Continued Care: Athletic activity usually can be resumed after an attack of cramps. If soreness persists, stop the activity and massage the muscle or use a heating pad to relax it.

Medication: Take aspirin, ibuprofen, or acetaminophen to help relieve pain and inflammation.

SPORTS FIRST AID

Long-Term Effects of Injury: None, with proper treatment.

Prevention of Recurring Injury: Add foods to your diet that are high in potassium and calcium: bananas, high-fiber cereals or bread, fresh vegetables, milk, yogurt, and cheese. Drink plenty of water before and during extended sporting events to help prevent muscle cramps from occurring. (Water helps the muscles eliminate waste products and helps you avoid dehydration.) In some instances—engaging in sports during hot weather, for example, when the body may be working twice as hard—cramping may occur even when precautionary measures have been taken.

See Your Physician: If muscle cramps occur regularly with athletic activity.

SHOULDER

Shoulder Dislocation (Instability)

What the Shoulder Is: The shoulder is a complex ball-and-socket-like joint consisting of three main bones—the humerus (the upper part of the upper arm bone), the clavicle (the collarbone), and the scapula (or shoulder blade, the largest bone in the chest-shoulder region). The humerus forms the ball in the ball-and-socket-like joint and is attached by ligaments—connective tissue—to the scapula.

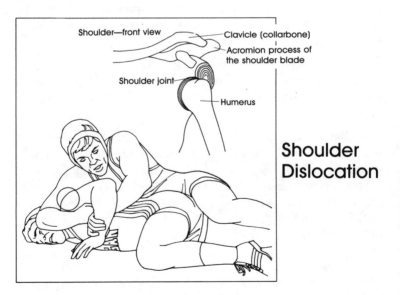

Shoulder—front view — Clavicle (collarbone)
— Acromion process of the shoulder blade
Shoulder joint —
— Humerus

Shoulder Dislocation

A dislocated shoulder is a shoulder "out of joint," caused by a fall or a direct blow to the shoulder region.

Bursas—fluid-filled sacs or saclike cavities—surround and cushion the bones and allow for movement. Muscles, including the trapezius, deltoid, pectorals, and latissimus dorsi, travel over, under, and around the shoulder joint and add stability. Tendons (also connective tissue) connect these muscles to bone.

What the Shoulder Does: The shoulder allows movement of the hand and arm in space.

What the Injury Is: A dislocated shoulder is a shoulder "out of joint." It occurs when the humeral bone in the upper arm comes out of the joint and sticks out, usually on the front or top of the shoulder. In severe cases, ligaments, tendons, and other connective tissues are stretched and injure nerves and blood vessels in the shoulder region, sometimes causing numbness in the hand.

Cause: The injury can be caused by a traumatic event, as in a direct blow to or a fall on the shoulder, or by a fall on your outstretched hand or arm. Susceptibility to a dislocation may also be genetic, particularly if the shoulder "goes out" or "pops out" often or easily. Members of the same family may also be afflicted. In some cases, the shoulder can dislocate while the individual is sleeping. A shoulder dislocation is common in contact sports, especially football. Other sports that may cause the injury: downhill skiing, lacrosse, hockey, volleyball, rugby, and soccer.

Symptoms: Severe pain at the moment the injury occurs. Limited movement in the shoulder area. Swelling, bruising, and internal bleeding. The shoulder may look odd, with a large bump rising up under the skin.

Immediate Treatment: Use an ice pack to reduce swelling. *Cold* treatments help stop internal bleeding and the accumulation of fluids in and around the injured area, thus decreasing swelling.

Seek medical treatment at a physician's office or hospital emergency room. (Individuals with recurring dislocations may be able to "pop" the shoulder back into place.) The shoulder may be put in a sling or wrapped to immobilize the area and aid recovery.

Medication: First, follow your physician's advice. You may be given a pain-relieving drug, such as codeine with aspirin or acetaminophen. You may also be given a nonsteroidal anti-inflammatory drug (NSAID) to reduce pain and swelling.

WARNING: *Do not give aspirin to children under the age of 16. If pregnant or nursing, consult with your physician first before taking any medication.*

Continued Care: Avoid participation in sports until the shoulder has had time to heal. The healing process may take 3 to 6 weeks, depending upon the extent of the injury. With your physician's okay, work with a trainer or physical therapist to strengthen muscles in the shoulder region.

Medication: First, follow the advice of your physician. Take aspirin, ibuprofen, or acetaminophen to help reduce pain and inflammation.

NOTE: *Acetaminophen may not contain as much of the anti-inflammatory agents as aspirin or ibuprofen. Ask your physician or pharmacist for guidance.*

Long-Term Effects of Injury: With proper healing, a full range of motion should return. In some cases, surgery may be recommended to help stabilize the shoulder. The procedure may involve cutting stretched ligaments and tendons.

Prevention of Recurring Injury: Avoid situations in which another injury could occur. Wear layers of clothing or padding to help cushion any fall that may be likely. Use weights and exercises advised by a trainer or physical therapist to strengthen muscles in the shoulder region. Muscle-strengthening exercises also help strengthen ligaments and tendons. Use an ice pack to reduce any swelling, then a heating pad to aid recovery. (*Heat* treatments help to enlarge the small blood vessels in and around the injured area, thus increasing blood circulation.)

See Your Physician: The first time a dislocation occurs, for rehabilitation and treatment to prevent recurrence.

Shoulder Separation

What the Shoulder Is: The shoulder is a complex ball-and-socket-like joint consisting of three main bones—the humerus (the upper part of the upper arm bone), the clavicle (the collarbone), and the scapula (or shoulder blade, the largest bone in the chest-shoulder region). The humerus forms the ball in the ball-and-socket-like joint and is attached by ligaments—connective tissue—to the scapula. Bursas—fluid-filled sacs or saclike cavities—surround and cushion the bones and allow for movement. Muscles, including the trapezius, deltoid, pectorals, and latissimus dorsi, travel over, under, and around the shoulder joint and add stability. Tendons (also connective tissue) connect these muscles to bone.

What the Shoulder Does: The shoulder allows movement of the hand and arm in space.

What the Injury Is: A shoulder separation occurs when ligaments that hold the collarbone to the shoulder blade are torn. The collarbone also may be pushed out of alignment.

Cause: The injury occurs from a traumatic event, as in a blow to or a fall on the shoulder area. It can also result from falling on your outstretched hand or arm. It is very common in contact sports, especially football. Other sports in which the injury may occur: downhill skiing, lacrosse, hockey, volleyball, rugby, and soccer.

Shoulder Separation

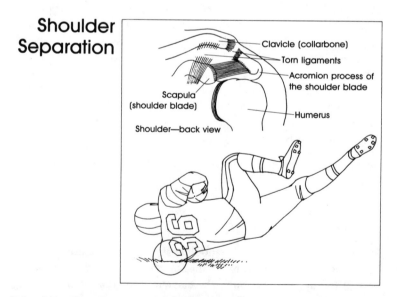

- Clavicle (collarbone)
- Torn ligaments
- Acromion process of the shoulder blade
- Humerus

Scapula (shoulder blade)

Shoulder—back view

A shoulder separation occurs when ligaments that hold the clavicle (collarbone) to the scapula (shoulder blade) are torn.

Symptoms: Severe pain at the moment the injury occurs. Limited movement in the shoulder area. Swelling, bruising, and internal bleeding. The shoulder may look malformed.

Immediate Treatment: Use an ice pack, if possible, as soon as the injury occurs. *Cold* treatments help stop internal bleeding and the accumulation of fluids in and around the injured area, thus decreasing swelling.

Seek medical treatment at a physician's office or hospital emergency room at once. *The injury should not be treated without professional medical attention.*

The shoulder will be put in a sling or wrapped to immobilize the area and aid recovery.

Medication: First, follow the advice of your physician. You may be given a pain-relieving drug, such as codeine with aspirin or acetaminophen. You may also be given a nonsteroidal anti-inflammatory drug (NSAID) to reduce pain and swelling.

WARNING: *Do not give aspirin to children under the age of 16. If pregnant or nursing, consult with your physician first before taking any medication.*

Continued Care: Avoid participation in sports until the injury has healed. Depending on its severity, the injury may take 2 to 10 weeks to heal. With your physician's okay, work with a trainer or physical therapist to strengthen muscles in the shoulder region.

Medication: First, follow your physician's advice. Take aspirin, ibuprofen, or acetaminophen to help reduce pain and inflammation.

NOTE: *Acetaminophen may not contain as much of the anti-inflammatory agents as aspirin or ibuprofen. Ask your physician or pharmacist for guidance.*

Long-Term Effects of Injury: There may be no lasting effects from the injury. In some individuals, however, stiffness or limitation of motion in the shoulder area may occur. In severe cases, surgery may be necessary to remove damaged tissue and to repair ligaments.

Prevention of Recurring Injury: Avoid situations in which another injury could occur. Wear layers of clothing or padding to help cushion any fall that may be likely. Use weights and exercises advised by a trainer or physical therapist to strengthen muscles in the

SPORTS FIRST AID

shoulder region. Muscle-strengthening exercises also help strengthen ligaments and tendons. Use an ice pack to reduce swelling, then a heating pad to aid recovery. (*Heat* treatments help to enlarge the small blood vessels in and around the injured area, thus increasing blood circulation.)

See Your Physician: If pain and swelling reappear and limit motion in the shoulder.

Swimmer's Shoulder

What the Shoulder Is: The shoulder is a complex ball-and-socket-like joint consisting of three main bones—the humerus (the upper part of the upper arm bone), the clavicle (the collarbone), and the scapula (or shoulder blade, the largest bone in the chest-shoulder region). The humerus forms the ball in the ball-and-socket-like joint and is attached by ligaments—connective tissue—to the scapula. Bursas—fluid-filled sacs or saclike cavities—surround and cushion

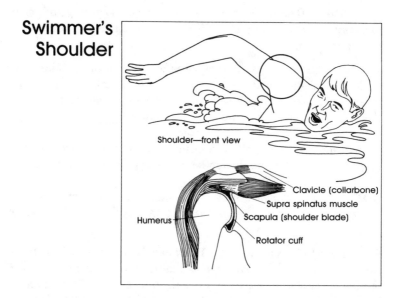

Swimmer's
Shoulder

Shoulder—front view

Clavicle (collarbone)
Supra spinatus muscle
Humerus
Scapula (shoulder blade)
Rotator cuff

Swimmer's shoulder is a strain and, sometimes, a microtear in the supraspinatus muscle. It can also be a strain or tear, called impingement syndrome, in the rotator cuff.

the bones and allow for movement. Muscles, including the trapezius, deltoid, pectorals, and latissimus dorsi, travel over, under, and around the shoulder joint and add stability. Tendons (also connective tissue) connect these muscles to bone.

What the Shoulder Does: The shoulder allows movement of the hand and arm in space.

What the Injury Is: Swimmer's shoulder is a strain and, sometimes, a microtear, in the supraspinatus muscle that lies on top of the shoulder between the neck and the top of the arm. It also can be a strain or tear, called an impingement syndrome, in the rotator cuff—an intertwined unit of muscles and tendons that surrounds and gives stability to the shoulder at the ball-socket joint. When trauma occurs to the rotator cuff, it may swell and "impinge" upon or rub against bone, causing pain.

Cause of Injury: The injury is usually associated with a repetitive motion over time. In swimming it also can be caused by an increase in distance or speed, or both, or by an improper swimming stroke. Other sports that can cause swimmer's shoulder: the baseball pitch, the football pass, the tennis serve, racquetball, volleyball, basketball, golf, sailing, canoeing, kayaking, javelin throw, shot put, weight lifting, and rock climbing. Other activities that may cause swimmer's shoulder: construction work, factory work, and other kinds of manual labor (painting, plastering, or housework); any prolonged activity in which the arm is extended above the head.

Symptoms: Pain on top and in the front of the shoulder. Pain in the shoulder at night. Pain and weakness when extending the arm forward or upward. You may feel as if you have a painful "hitch" in the shoulder. Sharp pain and limitation of motion in the shoulder joint (rotator cuff).

Immediate Treatment: *If the arm cannot be extended above the head, if the arm cannot be moved at all ("frozen shoulder"), or if there is a sharp pain and weakness where the arm connects to the trunk of the body, see your physician to determine proper treatment.* Stop the activity that is causing the pain. Place an ice pack on the shoulder as soon as possible. *Cold* treatments help stop internal bleeding and the accumulation of fluids in and around the injured area, thus decreasing swelling.

SPORTS FIRST AID

Medication: (If you have seen your physician, follow his or her advice.) Take aspirin, ibuprofen, or acetaminophen regularly to relieve pain and inflammation. Your physician may prescribe another mild analgesic (pain reliever) to help reduce pain or a nonsteroidal anti-inflammatory drug (NSAID) to help reduce pain and swelling. In some instances, your physician may suggest a low-dose injection of a corticosteroid or "steroid" drug, such as cortisone, that will help reduce inflammation.

NOTE: *Acetaminophen may not contain as much of the anti-inflammatory agents as aspirin or ibuprofen. Ask your physician or pharmacist for guidance.*

WARNING: *Do not give aspirin to children under the age of 16. If pregnant or nursing, consult with your physician first before taking any medication.*

Continued Care: Rest the arm for approximately 4 to 8 weeks. Use an ice pack for 2 to 4 days after ceasing the activity to reduce swelling and inflammation. Use a heating pad thereafter. *Heat* treatments help to enlarge the small blood vessels in and around the injured area, thus increasing blood circulation. (Blood carries vital nutrients to the injury and helps speed recovery.)

NOTE: *Heat should be applied only after swelling has subsided, or swelling in the injured area may increase.*

Do not engage in original activity until the pain has subsided. Ease into limited muscle workouts: gradually swing your arm as if throwing a ball, work with light weights, and work with a trainer or physical therapist on light shoulder exercises that use and strengthen the supraspinatus muscle. Use an ice pack to help reduce any swelling that may recur, then a heating pad to help repair the injury.

Medication: Take aspirin, ibuprofen, or acetaminophen to help reduce pain and inflammation.

Long-Term Effects of Injury: None, with proper treatment and rest, although some individuals may suffer recurring pain even with precautionary measures (see below). In rare cases, surgery may be recommended to remove scar tissue and bone from the rotator cuff area.

Prevention of Recurring Injury: Allow plenty of time for healing. Use weights and exercises advised by a trainer or physical therapist. These measures may have to be employed throughout a lifetime to avoid or reduce pain. Obtain the advice of a swimming instructor or baseball or football coach on proper technique.

Use an ice pack to reduce swelling, then a heating pad to aid recovery.

See Your Physician: If pain continues, is severe, or limits motion in the shoulder.

Medical Chart

Family Members (Names)	Allergies	DPT (DATE)	Tetanus Booster (DATE)	Measles (DATE)	Mumps (DATE)
Father					
Mother					
Children/Other					

Rubella (DATE)	Polio (DATE)	Influenza (Flu) (DATE)	Major Medical Problems (DATE)	Medications (DATES)	Other Medical Information

INDEX

ABC (airway, breathing, circulation), 19, 35
abdomen:
   description of, 53
   wounds in, 257–58
abdominal pain, 53–58
   in appendicitis, 53–54
   in bowel obstructions, 54–55
   in children, 57–58
   in ectopic pregnancy, 55–56
   in food poisoning, 184–85
   in gallbladder inflammations, 56
   in infants, 57–58
   in intussusception, 58
   in kidney stones, 56–57
   in malrotation, 57
   in menstrual cramps, 55
   in pancreatitis, 57
   in pyloric stenosis, 58
   in strangulated hernias, 58
abdominal thrust, see Heimlich maneuver
abuse victims, 115–18
accidents, safeguarding against:
   in basement, 7
   on basement stairs, 7
   in bathroom, 6–7
   in garage, 7
   in home, 6–7
   in kitchen, 6
achilles tendinitis, 300–302
acids, poisoning from, 217
acquired immune deficiency syndrome
   (AIDS):
   CPR administration and risk of, 18n
   in treating bleeding injuries, 80n–81n
adhesive strips, narrow, 42–43
adults:
   CPR on, 23–26
   diarrhea in, 144–45
   fevers in, 177–78
   Heimlich maneuver on, 37–39, 127–31
afterbirth, delivery of, 124
AIDS, see acquired immune deficiency
   syndrome
airway, breathing, circulation (ABC), 19, 35
airway obstructions, upper:
   breathing problems in, 90–92
   Heimlich maneuver for, 91–92
alcohol:
   abuse of, 156–57
   overdoses of, 156–57
   withdrawal from, 157
alkalis, poisoning from, 217
allergic reactions:
   to food, 234–35
   to insect stings, 65–67, 226, 234–37
   to medication, 234–35

altitude sickness, 59–60
ambulance services, 9–10
anaphylactic shock, 234–37
animal bites, 63
ankle injuries:
   broken bones, 96
   figure-of-eight bandages for, 44–45
   in sporting activities, 280–82
   sprains, 243, 280–82
appendicitis, abdominal pain in, 53–54
appetite loss:
   in appendicitis, 54
   in drug abuse, 158
   in gallbladder inflammations, 56
   in Rocky Mountain spotted fever, 229
arm injuries, broken bones, 96–98, 103–4
asthma, 61–62
avulsed teeth (knocked-out teeth), 140–41

back injuries:
   broken bones, 99–102
   in drowning victims, 149
   low back pain in, 267–69
   mouth-to-mouth resuscitation for, 100
   unconscious victims of, 101–2
bandages, 42–49
   butterfly, 42–43
   circular, 43–44
   cravat, 48–49
   figure-of-eight, 44–45
   fingertip, 45–46
   head, 48–49
   necktie, 48–49
   rectangular, 42
   roller gauze, 43–46
   scarf, 48–49
   triangular, 46–49
baseball finger (mallet finger), 285–86
basements, safeguarding against accidents in,
   7
basement stairs, safeguarding against
   accidents on, 7
bathrooms, safeguarding against accidents
   in, 6–7
bites:
   by animals, 63
   by humans, 64
   rashes from, 226
   by snakes, see snakebites
   by spiders, see spider bites
black eyes, 170
black widow spider bites, 68–69
bleeding, 80–86
   from cuts, 260–61
   direct pressure for, 80–82
   from ears, 162

drugs, therapeutic:
for achilles tendinitis, 301–2
allergic reactions to, 234–35
for baseball finger, 286
for gamekeeper's thumb, 288
for golfer's elbow, 271–72
for hamstring muscle pulls, 304–5
for heel spurs, 279–80
for hip pointers, 290
for low back pain, 268–69
for Morton's neuroma, 277–78
for muscle cramps, 309
for plantar fasciitis, 279–80
rashes from, 226–27
for runner's knee, 294
for shin splints, 306–7
for shoulder dislocations, 312–13
for shoulder separations, 315
for skier's thumb, 288
for sprained ankles, 282
for stress fractures, 284
for swimmer's shoulder, 318
for tennis elbow, 274–75
for torn cartilage in knees, 296–97
for torn ligaments in knees, 299

earaches, 163
ear injuries, 162–65
bleeding in, 162
foreign objects in, 163–64
frostbite in, 164–65
ECG (electrocardiographic) tracings, 9
ectopic pregnancy, abdominal pain in, 55–56
elbow injuries:
broken bones, 103–4
golfer's elbow, 270–73
in sporting activities, 270–75
sprains, 244
tennis elbow, 273–75
electric shock, 166–68
mouth-to-mouth resuscitation for victims
of, 168
electrocardiographic (ECG) tracings, 9
emergencies:
in childbirth, see childbirth emergencies
dental, see dental emergencies
everyday items used in, 5
immediate treatments for, i
preparing for, 3–5
supplies to keep in home and car for, 4–5
telephone numbers in, ii
what to do in, i
what to tell doctors or paramedics in, i
emergency kits for insect stings, 237
emergency medical identification bracelets,
3–4
emergency medical technician (EMT)
paramedics, 9
emergency rooms:
information to give personnel in, 10–11
when to go to, 10
epiglottitis, breathing problems in, 89–90
epileptic seizures, 136

exhaustion, heat, 210
external bleeding, 80–85
direct pressure for, 80–82
pressure points for, 82–83
tourniquets for, 83–84
extractions (pulled teeth), 141
extremities:
loss of motion in, 17
loss of sensation in, 17
severed, 232–33
see also foot injuries; hand injuries
eye infections, 171–72
chalazion, 171
conjunctivitis, 171
pinkeye, 171
styes, 171–72
eye injuries, 17, 169–74
black eyes, 170
blunt, 170
chemical burns, 169–70
contact lenses in victims of, 172
cuts, 172
flushing out eyes in, 170
foreign bodies in, 172–74
and removal of foreign bodies, 174
eyes:
changes in sizes of pupils of, 14–15
normal pupils in, 14–15

Fahrenheit thermometers, 13, 179
fainting, 175–76
family members:
familiarity with state of health of, 12–17
medical charts for, 3, 320–21
pulse rates of, 13–14
pupil sizes of, 14–15
temperatures of, 12–13
fatigue, 268–69
fevers, 15, 177–80
in adults, 177–78
in appendicitis, 54
in asthma, 61
in children, 178–80
in croup, 88
diarrhea and, 146
in drug abuse, 157, 159
in food poisoning, 185
in gallbladder inflammations, 56
in infants, 178–80
in lead poisoning, 200
in Lyme disease, 204
multiple insect stings and, 67
of 105° F., 211
in overexposure, 211
in plant irritations, 215
in pregnancy, 221
in Rocky Mountain spotted fever, 229
in shock, 240–41
spider bites and, 70
fiddleback spider (brown recluse spider)
bites, 69–70
figure-of-eight bandages, 44–45
finger injuries, bandages for, 43–46

fingertip bandages, 45–46
fingertip injuries (hammer-hit injuries;
    door-crush injuries), 181
first aid:
  bandages in, 42–49
  butterfly bandages in, 42–43
  circular bandages in, 43–44
  cravat bandages in, 48–49
  dressings in, 41
  figure-of-eight bandages in, 44–45
  fingertip bandages in, 45–46
  head bandages in, 48–49
  narrow adhesive strips in, 42–43
  necktie bandages in, 48–49
  rectangular bandages in, 42
  roller gauze bandages in, 43–46
  scarf bandages in, 48–49
  slings in, 47
  splints in, *see* splints
  for sports injuries, 265–319
  techniques in, 41–49
  triangular bandages in, 46–49
first-degree burns, 109–10
fishhook injuries, 182
food, allergic reactions to, 234–35
food poisoning, 183–85
  botulism in, 183
  from mushrooms, 183–84
  from salmonella, 184–85
  from staphylococcus, 185
foot injuries:
  ankle sprains, 243, 280–82
  heel spurs, 278–80
  Morton's neuroma, 276–78
  plantar fasciitis, 278–80
  in sporting activities, 276–84
  stress fractures, 283–84
foreign bodies:
  in ears, 163–64
  inside eyelids, 173–74
  in eyes, 172–74
  floating on eyeballs, 173–74
  removal from eyes of, 174
  resting on eyeballs, 173–74
  sticking into eyeballs, 173
fractures, *see* broken bones
freezing in hypothermia, 214
frostbite, 212–13
  in ears, 164–65
fumes, poisoning from, 186

gallbladder inflammations, abdominal pain
    in, 56
gamekeeper's thumb (skier's thumb),
    287–88
garages, safeguarding against accidents in, 7
gas leaks, poisoning from, 186
gauze bandages, 43–46
golfer's elbow, 270–73

hallucinogens:
  abuse of, 159–60
  overdoses of, 159–60

hammer-hit injuries (fingertip injuries;
    door-crush injuries), 181
hamstring muscle pulls, 302–5
hand injuries:
  baseball finger, 285–86
  broken bones, 104
  figure-of-eight bandages for, 44–45
  gamekeeper's thumb, 287–88
  mallet finger, 285–86
  skier's thumb, 287–88
  in sporting activities, 285–88
hand position for CPR, 24, 28–29
head, location of pressure points on, 83
headaches, 15–16, 187
  in altitude sickness, 59
  in food poisoning, 183, 185
  in head injuries, 188
  in Lyme disease, 204
  multiple insect stings and, 67
  in neck injuries, 191
  in overexposure, 210
  in plant irritations, 215
  in pregnancy, 187, 221
  in Rocky Mountain spotted fever, 229
  severe, 16–17
  in strokes, 246
head bandages, 48–49
head injuries, 188–91, 194–95
  broken bones, 195
  mouth-to-mouth resuscitation in, 189
  moving victims of, 194
  scalp cuts, 195
  triangular bandages for, 46–49
heart attacks, 196–98
  in conscious victims, 198
  mouth-to-mouth resuscitation in,
    197
  in self, 198
  in unconscious victims who are not
    breathing, 196–97
heat injuries, 209–12
  cramps in, 209–10
  exhaustion in, 210
  heatstroke in, 210–11
  sunburn in, 211–12
  sunstroke in, 210–11
heat rashes (prickly heat), 227
heel spurs (plantar fasciitis), 278–80
Heimlich maneuver (abdominal thrust):
  on adults, 37–39, 127–30
  on children, 37–39, 91–92, 127–32
  for choking, 18, 36–40, 91–92, 127–32
  on conscious victims, 37–38, 127–30
  on infants, 39–40, 92, 131
  in life and death situations, 18, 36–40
  during pregnancy, 40, 132
  on reclining victims, 38, 130–31
  on self, 40, 132
  on unconscious victims, 38–39, 130–31
  for upper airway obstructions, 91–92
  on very fat victims, 40, 132
hernias, strangulated (incarcerated), 58

for victims who are not breathing, 21, 197
for wounds, 259
multiple stings (toxic reaction), 67–68
muscle injuries:
  aches and pains in, 208
  cramps, 308–10
  hamstring pulls, 302–5
  low back pain in, 267–69
  pulls, 267–69, 302–5
  in sporting activities, 302–5, 308–10
  strains, 245
  tears, 267–69
mushroom poisoning, 183–84

National Safety Council, 6
nausea, 15
  in allergic reactions to insect stings, 65
  in altitude sickness, 59
  in appendicitis, 54
  in bowel obstructions, 54
  in diabetic comas, 142
  in drug abuse, 157
  in fainting, 175
  in food poisoning, 185
  in gallbladder inflammations, 56
  in heart attacks, 196
  kidney stones and, 56
  marine life stings and, 71
  in overexposure, 210
  in pancreatitis, 57
  scorpion stings and, 72
  in shock, 234
  snakebites and, 75, 79
  spider bites and, 68, 70
  in vertigo, 254
neck injuries, 191–94
  broken bones, 193
  in drowning victims, 149
  immobilization for, 193
  mouth-to-mouth resuscitation in, 189
  moving victims of, 191–92, 194
necktie bandages, 48–49
newborns:
  emergency delivery of, 121–22
  post-delivery care for, 122–23
  preparations prior to arrival of, 119–20
  tying umbilical cords of, 123–24
  see also infants
nonpoisonous snakebites, 79
nosebleeds, 86

open fractures, 93
open wounds, 257–63
  in abdomen, 257–58
  in chest, 258–60
  from cuts, 260–61
  mouth-to-mouth resuscitation for victims of, 259
  from punctures, 262–63
  from scrapes and scratches, 263
overdoses:
  of alcohol, 156–57

of depressants, 158
of hallucinogens, 159–60
of stimulants, 160–61
overexposure, 209–14
  cold injuries from, 164–65, 212–14
  frostbite from, 164–65, 212–13
  heat cramps from, 209–10
  heat exhaustion from, 210
  heat injuries from, 209–12
  heatstroke from, 210–11
  hypothermia from, 214
  mild chilling from, 214
  sunburn from, 211–12
  sunstroke from, 210–11

pains:
  abdominal, see abdominal pain
  in abuse victims, 115
  in achilles tendinitis, 301
  in baseball finger, 286
  in broken bones, 93, 284
  in bruises, 108
  in burns, 110–11
  in chest, see chest pain
  in closed wounds, 264
  in decompression sickness, 138
  in dislocations, 147
  in ear injuries, 162–64
  in forefoot, 276–78
  in golfer's elbow, 271
  in hamstring muscle tears, 303
  in heel spurs, 279
  in hip pointers, 290
  in insect stings, 64
  in kidney stones, 56–57
  in knee cartilage tears, 296
  in knee ligament tears, 298
  in low back, 267–69
  in marine life stings, 71
  in muscle cramps, 309
  in muscles, 208
  in overexposure, 209, 211–12
  in plantar fasciitis, 279
  in pregnancy, 221
  in runner's knee, 293
  in scorpion stings, 72
  in sexual assault, 222
  in shin splints, 306
  in shoulder dislocations, 312
  in shoulder separations, 315
  in skier's thumb, 288
  in snakebites, 75, 79
  in spider bites, 68, 70
  in sprains, 243, 281
  in stress fractures, 284
  in swimmer's shoulder, 317
  in tennis elbow, 274
pancreatitis, abdominal pain in, 57
paramedics:
  ambulance services and, 9–10
  in emergencies, i
  EMT, 9
pelvis injuries, broken bones, 107

petroleum products, poisoning from, 217
pinkeye (conjunctivitis), 171
plantar fasciitis (heel spurs), 278–80
plant irritations, 215, 227
poisoning, 216–20
   from acids, 217
   from alkalis, 217
   botulism in, 183
   in conscious victims, 218–20
   convulsions in, 200, 218
   from food, 183–85
   from fumes, 186
   from gas leaks, 186
   from lead, 200
   mouth-to-mouth resuscitation for, 219
   from mushrooms, 183–84
   from petroleum products, 217
   from salmonella, 184–85
   from staphylococcus, 185
   in unconscious victims, 218
   in victims who are not breathing, 217
poison ivy, 215
poison oak, 215
poisonous rashes, 215, 227
poisonous snakes:
   characteristics of, 75
   triangular-shaped heads of, 75
   see also snakebites
poison sumac, 215
Portuguese-man-of-war stings, 71–72
pregnancy:
   danger signs in, 221
   ectopic, 55–56
   headaches during, 187, 221
   Heimlich maneuver during, 40, 132
   miscarriages and, 207
   see also childbirth emergencies
pressure, direct, for bleeding, 80–82
pressure points:
   for bleeding, 82–83
   location of, 83
prickly heat (heat rashes), 227
projectile vomiting, 58
psychogenic shock, 239–40
pulled teeth (extractions), 141
pulse rates:
   CPR and, 23–24, 27, 31, 35
   of family members, 13–14
   how to find, 13–14, 23, 27, 31
   meaning of, 35
   normal, 13–14
puncture wounds, 262–63
pupils of eyes:
   changes in sizes of, 14–15
   of family members, 14–15
   normal, 14–15
pyloric stenosis, abdominal pain in, 58

rape, 222–25
   continued care for, 225
   dos and don'ts for, 223
   immediate treatment for, 223

mouth-to-mouth resuscitation for victims
   of, 224
symptoms of, 222
rashes, 226–28
   in allergic reactions to insect stings, 65, 226
   from bites, 226
   diaper, 227–228
   from diseases, 226
   from drugs, 226–27
   from heat, 227
   hives, 227
   in infants, 227–228
   poisonous, 215, 227
rattlesnake bites, 66, 73–78
reclining victims, Heimlich maneuver on, 38, 130–31
rectangular bandages, 42
respiration, 35
resuscitation:
   meaning of, 35–36
   see also cardiopulmonary resuscitation;
      mouth-to-mouth resuscitation
Rocky Mountain spotted fever, 229–31
   prevention of, 230–31
roller gauze bandages, 43–46
runner's knee, 292–95

salmonella poisoning, 184–85
salt-and-sugar-water solutions, 146
scalp cuts, 195
scarf bandages, 48–49
scorpion stings, 72–73
scrapes, 263
scratches, 263
second-degree burns, 110–11, 113
seizures, see convulsions
sensation, loss of, 17
separations, shoulder, 313–16
septic shock, 240
severe bleeding, 260–61
severe chest pain, 17
severed limbs, 232–33
severe headaches, 16–17
sexual abuse, 115–18
   dos and don'ts for, 118
   mouth-to-mouth resuscitation for, 117
sexual assault, 222–25
   continued care for, 225
   dos and don'ts for, 223
   immediate treatment for, 223
   mouth-to-mouth resuscitation for victims
      of, 224
   symptoms of, 222
shallow water blackouts, 152–53
shin splints, 305–7
shock, 234–41
   anaphylactic, 234–37
   insulin, 239
   psychogenic, 239–40
   septic, 240
   toxic, 240–41
   traumatic, 237–39

shoulder injuries:
  broken bones, 107
  dislocations, 311–13
  separations, 313–16
  in sporting activities, 311–19
  sprains, 244
  swimmer's shoulder, 316–19
skier's thumb (gamekeeper's thumb),
    287–88
skull fractures, 195
slings, 47
snakebites, 73–79
  by copperheads, 66, 73, 75–78
  by coral snakes, 73–74, 78–79
  by cottonmouthes, 66, 73–78
  nonpoisonous, 79
  poisonous, 66, 73–79
  by rattlesnakes, 66, 73–78
  removing venom after, 77–78
  tourniquets for, 66, 76–77
spider bites, 68–71
  by black widow spiders, 68–69
  by brown recluse spiders, 69–70
  by tarantulas, 70–71
spinal injuries, see back injuries; neck
    injuries
splinters, 242
splints, 49
  for ankles, 96
  for broken bones, 95–98, 104–7
  for hand injuries, 104
  for kneecap injuries, 104–5
  for lower arm injuries, 98
  for lower leg injuries, 106–7
  for upper arm injuries, 96–97
  for upper leg injuries, 105–6
  for wrists, 98
sports injuries, 265–319
  achilles tendinitis, 300–302
  to back, 267–69
  baseball finger, 285–86
  to elbows, 270–75
  to feet, 276–84
  gamekeeper's thumb, 287–88
  golfer's elbow, 270–73
  hamstring muscle pulls, 302–5
  to hands, 285–88
  heel spurs, 278–80
  hip pointers, 289–91
  to knees, 292–99
  to legs, 300–307
  low back pain, 267–69
  mallet finger, 285–86
  Morton's neuroma, 276–78
  muscle cramps, 308–10
  to muscles, 302–5, 308–10
  plantar fasciitis, 278–80
  runner's knee, 292–95
  shin splints, 305–7
  shoulder dislocations, 311–13
  to shoulders, 311–19
  shoulder separations, 313–16
  skier's thumb, 287–88

sprained ankles, 280–82
stress fractures, 283–84
swimmer's shoulder, 316–19
tennis elbow, 273–75
torn cartilage in knees, 295–97
torn ligaments in knees, 297–99
sprains, 243–44
  of ankles, 243, 280–82
  of elbows, 244
  of knees, 243
  of shoulders, 244
  of wrists, 244
staphylococcus poisoning, 185
stiffness, 268–69
stimulants:
  abuse of, 160–61
  overdoses of, 160–61
  withdrawal from, 161
stings:
  by insects, see insect stings
  by marine life, 71–72
  rashes from, 65, 226
  by scorpions, 72–73
stools:
  blood in, 17, 85, 144, 146, 264
  in diarrhea, 144–45
strangulated (incarcerated) hernias,
    abdominal pain in, 58
stress fractures in sporting activities, 283–84
strokes, 246–48
  major, 246–48
  minor, 248
  mouth-to-mouth resuscitation for victims
    of, 247
  TIAs, 248
styes, 171–72
suicides, threatened, 249–50
sunburn, 211–12
sunstroke (heatstroke), 210–11
swimmer's shoulder, 316–19

tape (butterfly bandages), 42–43
tarantula bites, 70–71
teeth, see dental emergencies
telephone numbers, emergency, ii
temperatures:
  of family members, 12–13
  high, see fevers
  how to take, 179–80
  normal, 12
tendinitis, achilles, 300–302
tennis elbow, 273–75
thermometers, 13
  Celsius, 13, 179
  Fahrenheit, 13, 179
  how to read, 178–79
thigh (upper leg) injuries, broken bones,
    105–6
third-degree burns, 111–14
threatened suicides, 249–50
TIAs (transient ischemic attacks), 248
ticks:
  Lyme disease carried by, 204–6

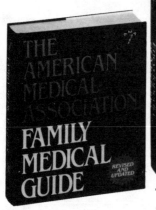
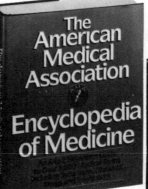
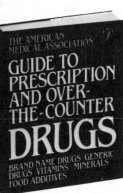